Prisoners of our Perceptions

Prisoners of our Perceptions

Medical Hypnoanalysis in Action

Dr. Trevor Modlin

Copyright © 2020 by Dr. Trevor Modlin.

Library of Congress Control Number:		2020901273
ISBN:	Hardcover	978-1-7960-8345-3
	Softcover	978-1-7960-8344-6
	eBook	978-1-7960-8343-9

All rights reserved. No part of this book may be reproduced or transmitted in any form or by any means, electronic or mechanical, including photocopying, recording, or by any information storage and retrieval system, without permission in writing from the copyright owner.

Any people depicted in stock imagery provided by Getty Images are models, and such images are being used for illustrative purposes only.
Certain stock imagery © Getty Images.

Print information available on the last page.

Rev. date: 01/17/2020

To order additional copies of this book, contact:
Xlibris
1-888-795-4274
www.Xlibris.com
Orders@Xlibris.com
808370

CONTENTS

Acknowledgements and Dedications ix
Introduction xi

Chapter 1   Migraine: The Light at the end of the tunnel 1
Chapter 2   Clinical Hypnosis 8
Chapter 3   Of Mind, Body and Spirit...27
Chapter 4   Psychosomatic Disease 41
Chapter 5   Medical Hypnoanalysis..57
Chapter 6   The Subconscious Diagnoses 66
Chapter 7   More on Diagnosis..80
Chapter 8   The Healing Process of Medical Hypnoanalysis...........96
Chapter 9   Case Histories : Asthma... 112
Chapter 10   Systemic Lupus Erythematosus 123
Chapter 11   Anorexia, Bulimia and Depression 137
Chapter 12   Depression 150
Chapter 13   Post-traumatic Stress Disorder 167
Chapter 14   Panic Disorder 176
Chapter 15   Myalgic Encephalomyelitis (ME) 186
Chapter 16   Habit Disorders 200
Chapter 17   Cocaine Addiction.. 216
Chapter 18   Personality Disorder..230
Chapter 19   Obsessive Compulsive Disorder (OCD) 242
Chapter 20   Cancer 250
Chapter 21   A Review ... and the Future....................................... 264

Sources, References and Glossary 275
Glossary 281

If you seek purposeful meaning
there are just six words in this universe which are of real importance
which need to be actualised.
Six words which can alter one's self from conflict to peace.

The words are:

I am alive ... and ... **I love me**

for there is no greater satisfaction than to generate,
magnify and give Love.

ACKNOWLEDGEMENTS AND DEDICATIONS

I have experienced a life full of many interesting people and events – some wonderfully satisfying and some very threatening. All of them contribute to Life in lessons learned and valued.

I give profound thanks to my nuclear and extended family, my teachers and friends all of whom played an important part in my life. I am particularly gratified with the personal and career achievements of my children Steve, Melissa and Roderick.

To patients everywhere, especially those who allowed me the privilege of helping them - and those I could not.

To my beloved Beverley, who has more Light, Love and Integrity than anyone I know - an exceptional human – and courage beyond the norm for risking marrying me! I love her and thank her for being; I thank her for the rewards of Loving.

I give thanks to the Light for providing me with the opportunity to have such a full and rewarding Life here.

Love and Light to you all.

INTRODUCTION

Mind is the Master Power that moulds and makes,
And Man is Mind;
And ever more he takes the tool of thought
And, shaping what he wills,
Brings forth a thousand joys, a thousand ills.

James Joyce

We have all been visitors to the 'dark place' – every one of us, at one or other time. Many remain trapped in that bleak void, resigned and without hope of ever seeing light once more. They have forgotten what it is to laugh, to live. They have lost their way, lost their connection.

If one had the time and resources to review medicine, psychiatry and psychology one would find one common theme - a theme integral to life itself: change. The pendulum has swung from the mind and life experiences to genetics and biochemistry. At present the latter holds sway, especially with the advent of drugs like the selective serotonin re-uptake inhibitors.

Yet today, exciting adventures in modern clinical hypnotherapy and epigenetics have again raised questions regarding the purely genetic and biochemical theory of disease, known as reductionist theory.

Utilising the subconscious mind's enormous resources, many patients - especially in the USA, in South Africa and more recently in Australia - have been able to understand that many of their problems were not always so, that their uncomfortable lot in life was due to the learned responses to apparently devastating events early in life ... and I do mean specifically 'early'! They have realised that they can unlearn these responses and ... change. There is ever hope. In the noble spiritual nature of humankind there is always a very special energy to be found at its source - love is the key which unlocks the barriers and the defences ...

love is the warm place in the heart ... the light which leads out of the 'dark place'.

I thought long and hard about committing the experiences of some of my patients to paper. It was not easy for many of them and I trust you, the reader, to respect and honour their pain while at the same time to share their triumphs. Their courage has been self-rewarding and they represent hope to others.

I practise medicine. Let there be no mistake about that. Drawing on more than five decades of study and practice, I practise the art of medicine. Yes, it is an art ... despite the bio-technology of modern times. However, in following this art all too often we forget the words of James Joyce. It is sad to record that medicine has, in many ways, lost the art of knowing the human spirit. This loss has been proportional to the rise of modern technological medicine.

Medical schools world-wide have a common problem in that they are obliged, as academic institutions, to provide their eager as well as their not so keen students with scientific knowledge. It is a daunting task which they carry out magnificently. I should know - while I was still in general practice I held an honorary lecturer's post in the Department of Family Medicine of my alma mater, the University of Witwatersrand. It was my privilege to see some of these students attached to my practice for a week at a time. The standard of their knowledge has not decreased, as so many people are ready to cry - quite the contrary. It was a humbling experience to interact with them.

Yet there are doctors who deny that they see, for example, depression in their practices. I am not being critical of doctors in general - most are compassionate and able people answering to their calling. Yet, pharmaceutical representatives have personally told me that, when detailing anti-depressant drugs, there are a few doctors who do deny that they see depression. And there are those who provide more destructive suggestions. A patient I saw was told by her GP "You're just a depressed person. Accept it." He was entirely dismissive of her problem, which encourages a defeatist attitude and guarantees the continuation of the depression. The message the patient receives is: "There's no hope, loser, so don't bother me with something I cannot help you with." Whatever hope and compassion the patient sought is summarily destroyed, and an unhealthy dose of guilt added at the same time. One wonders what conclusions many other people with chronic pain syndromes, rheumatoid arthritis, lupus and many other diseases have reached.

In twenty-five years of family and hospital practice I witnessed a great deal. Very often I experienced a gut feeling of more important factors below the surface of the presenting symptoms. It required a near catastrophe of my own to be able to stand back a little, to review some things. It gave me the opportunity to see what was there, underlying the morass of physical ills that was presented to me sometimes for eighteen hours a day.

For example, and I will discuss many others later, I did not see one patient with an overactive thyroid who did not have clinically significant anxiety within a few years before the thyroid gland began malfunctioning. Many of these patients did not recognise their own fears and a few vehemently denied them, to the extent of stomping angrily out of the rooms. This was before I knew of the term 'transference' - a phenomenon still so poorly taught to medical undergraduates. Transference, very simply, indicates the emotions which can be transferred from patient to doctor or *vice versa* - and these emotions can be good, positive ones ... or, very negative and destructive ones. It is not difficult to learn how to deal with transference and it would certainly obviate a great deal of suffering - from both the patients' point of view as well as the poor old general practitioners.

But we can and do learn. That is what we're here for, after all ... to raise every facet of our lives to higher levels – essentially to the ability to generate, magnify and give Love. And, usually, to learn we need to **change** some beliefs and we need a teacher. I had a great many teachers - from my lecturers at university, my revered registrars and chiefs when I was an intern, to all those patients who had the grace to bless me as their doctor and, sometimes, the courage to come and see me. I mean this quite literally ... and they know what I mean ... they trusted me.

There was one other colleague who taught me - a man with the courage to stand up and risk ridicule. I privately thought he'd lost the plot. But he had the last laugh because he was actually helping patients in a way that was fascinating to me though foreign to my thoroughly scientific training. The late Dr. Jules Leeb taught me clinical hypnosis, he taught me to open my eyes, to really listen and how to take positive action.

Many wonderful books have been written by exceptional people like Dr. Bernie Siegel, for example. I know they have been trying to share their work, to educate us about what is possible, to give us hope. Sadly, there are just as many books and articles published which are critical, which suggest that there are no cures, that one's genetic code determines all. I wonder how long we can afford to continue to ignore the obvious and obstruct a truly holistic approach and not the facile 'holisim' so often bandied about. Like the ignorant doctor and his depressed patient, do we preach that all hope should be abandoned? I suggest that one should **reject** those suggestions ... they are not truth. As you will see, we are indeed prisoners of our own perceptions and each of us has the power to change.

To those people who feel they need something further, consider what Dr Bernie Siegel wrote in his book **Love, Medicine and Miracles:** *"The process of restructuring your life, of becoming an authentic person means ceasing to think of yourself as a thing - a collection of habits, a job, a role. This is being a slave of your self-image and in a sense, already dead."*

As you will discover, being 'dead' is what we call the Walking Zombie Syndrome in Medical Hypnoanalysis. This 'self-image' is formed by perceptions of life's experiences from as early as the womb which become fixed in the subconscious.

To those clinicians who read this book, I quote liberally from an editorial in the **South African Medical Journal - Volume 86, Number 8** - written by ARP Walker of Witwatersrand University and the SA Institute for Medical Research and co-authored by D. Labadarios of the University of Stellenbosch: *"Long ago, Abelard urged 'The first key to wisdom is assiduous and frequent questioning ... For by doubting we come to enquiry, and by enquiring we come to the truth.'"*

Moses Maimonides was a physician and revered Jewish philosopher of the twelfth century. The above authors point out that he *"wrote of how the emotions of the soul involve great alterations in the body (functions)."*

They continue to add *"Sir William Osler (an acknowledged father of modern medicine) considered it more important to know the patient who has the disease than the kind of disease from which he is suffering."*

This book may be considered threatening by some - that is not my intent, rather I seek to challenge, to invite. Its primary purpose is to stimulate thought and provide hope. This book is about how I became involved in clinical hypnosis and one of its modern techniques - Medical Hypnoanalysis - which I have found to be so remarkably rewarding to so many patients that it warrants a wider exposure. The book is about our bodies, our minds, and most of all it is about the human spirit and faith. It is about patients of mine who had the courage to confront what they'd known all along, deep inside. It's a record of a new journey that more and more are following with just reward.

It is about what James Joyce had to say ... and every word of his is true.

CHAPTER ONE

Migraine: The Light at the end of the tunnel

The mind has its own womb to which, baffled by speculation, it longs to return.
Cyril Connolly: The Unquiet Grave, 1945.

John was 36 years old when he came to see me and had experienced migraine since he was about ten or eleven years old.

When asked what his problem was, he said: "I get migraines. I get this terrible stiffness in my neck then it comes over - usually in my right eye. It becomes throbbing. I get nausea. I can't handle light or noise. I retract, I go into myself with this pain - I can **suffer** with my pain, but it's affecting my family. I can't do my job. I can't communicate with people. I have to cut off from everything and everybody to come over this thing. Then I can get on with my life again".

Listening closely to his words and for you to read into them it is quite clear he was 'dead' and with the word 'suffer' there is an indication of guilt with self-punishment.

He had been on various types of medication to try and prevent the onset of migraine, with little success. To deal with the pain he had in the past taken pain killers and sleeping pills, as sleep helped him. He had seen specialists and been investigated with no pathological findings. The migraines occurred up to three times a week and were so immobilising that he could not function at work.

Further history revealed a generalised anxiety disorder, a dysthymic depression and other less troublesome problems. He said he had been an anxious person, "I think from birth."

He was his parents' first child and when asked about his mother's pregnancy with him and of his birth, he said: "It was traumatic for her; it was a long birth." During the pregnancy she had fainted a lot. His mother came from a very dysfunctional family and her father was often drunk and abusive. His own childhood was unhappy, with a strict father who used beatings to discipline the children, while his mother was a perfectionist. He had not felt loved as a child and recalled those years as being filled with anxiety and guilt. He considered himself a failure at school, not being able to please his parents or teachers. He had often been humiliated by them. He described his childhood as "something I would like to forget."

His assessment revealed that he probably had problems while still in the womb, a traumatic birth experience and an event at age ten or eleven which precipitated his migraine. There was likely to be guilt involved in this because of his statement "I can suffer with my pain, but it's affecting my family."

In his prenatal regression, he was taken to his mother's first awareness of the pregnancy.

John = patient
T = therapist

John : She knows I'm here. She's scared of the unknown.
T : How are you feeling?
John : Not wanted. She's not happy to be pregnant with me. She wants to love but she doesn't know how. I feel alone, not wanted.

At five months *in utero* :

T : Feel out for your mother and see if you're picking up anything from her.
John : She's tired and fainting a lot.
T : Does this affect you?

John	: Yes, I'm scared. She works hard.
T	: How do you feel about this?
John	: I'm responsible. If I wasn't here, she'd be better off.
T	: Are you aware of any meaning for yourself?
John	: No.
T	: How are you dealing with this?
John	: I have to fight. Stay alive.
T	: How? Are you angry?
John	: No. I can just be quiet and good, to help her.
T	: Physically, do you feel alive?
John	: Yes.
T	: Emotionally?
John	: I know I'm there.
T	: Spiritually?
John	: No.
T	: How does that make you feel?
John	: It's a dying feeling.

With these uncertain beginnings, his subconscious gave permission to experience the birth:

John	: I feel pressure on my feet - claustrophobic [begins to hyperventilate on and off]. My mother is scared.
T	: Are you moving?
John	: Yes.
T	: What part of you is going first?
John	: My head. It's tight. Very narrow. I'm scared I'm going to hurt her.
T	: What will happen?
John	: She might die...
T	: And you?

John	: No! I don't want her to die. I don't know ... I will die. Pain all over my head. My chest is tight. I want to breathe ... I can't breathe ...
T	: What does that mean to you?
John	: I will die. I'm scared. My heart's racing.
T	: Are you still moving?
John	: If I struggle it hurts my mom. I'm dizzy. Nausea. Confused. I must just be quiet ... It's **sore!**
T	: Where?
John	: My head. She's holding back. She doesn't want to let go. I will die. I want to kick. Cross and angry. I **got to get out**. There's no space - the doctor is screaming at her.
T	: Are you moving?
John	: No. I'm resting.
T	: For what reason?
John	: I'm exhausted ... **God it's sore!**
T	: Where?
John	: Around my head!

[He starts writhing and gasping].

John	: Head's getting cold. Somebody's touching me ... oh! it's sore ... they're pulling on my head!!

[John now holds his breath, becomes red in the face and turns his head to the side - which is the movement of the head as it is delivered].

John	: **I can breathe!** [panting]
T	: Take a **deep** breath ... hold it, hold it, hold it ... now slowly let it out ... good ... what does that breath tell you?
John	: I'm **alive!** I'm very tired. They're working on my mother. I'm cold. I'm **alone.** She's crying. I want to go back, in my mom.

T	: For what reason?
John	: I'll be safe and warm.
T	: Are you picking up on any love?
John	: No. I want to be with her.
T	: What do you think her reaction will be?
John	: I don't know. I'm worried.
T	: About?
John	: If she wants me.
T	: If she doesn't?
John	: It'll be terrible - it'll feel like dying.
T	: Go to that time you're with her.
John	: She's holding me. It's familiar. I can smell her. She's looking at me. She's very, very tired.
T	: Are you picking up on love?
John	: No. I don't care. I just want to be with her. They're taking me away.
T	: How do you feel about that?
John	: It's OK. They're showing me to my father.
T	: What do you pick up from him?
John	: Oh, love... lots of love.

Subsequently, he contacted his mother who confirmed that he had been a forceps delivery. The extreme pain of the pressure on his head before and especially when the forceps were applied was the same kind of pain he experienced with migraine. He came to realise that in 'pressure situations' he was responding with the **same feelings,** physically and emotionally, as his birth experience. His subconscious had assumed that, as he **had** survived, this was the manner in which to respond in order to survive any perceived threat, to 'get through' a crisis.

With conscious understanding of his survival, his migraines ceased.

However, this is not the whole story of his migraine. He experienced two or three events which intensified a feeling of not being wanted and which of course increased his perception of being unworthy and guilty. One such example, at the age of seven years:

John is at home, and very agitated.

T	: What is happening?
John	: I want to go away to Mrs Y [a neighbour].
T	: For what reason?
John	: My parents are fighting.
T	: How do you feel?
John	: I'm unhappy. Worried.
T	: What are you going to do?
John	: Want to **get out**! [the same survival compulsion of the birth experience].
T	: What is it you're scared of?
John	: I'm scared my dad will kill us. I'm very tense.
T	: What are they fighting about?
John	: I don't know. I feel responsible.
T	: What can you do?
John	: I can go away. They will be rid of me.
T	: How will that help?
John	: I'll feel better.

The Symptom Producing Event occurred at the age of eleven when he was baby-sitting his sister:

T	: Where are you?
John	: At home. My baby sister's been born. I'm looking after her.
T	: What is happening now?
John	: She's crying, screaming.
T	: What do you do?
John	: I can't do anything.
T	: How are you feeling?

John	: I feel responsible, scared. If my parents come home to this they'll be disappointed - it'll make me feel bad. She's sucking on my finger.
T	: What do you do?
John	: She must be hungry. She doesn't take the teat. **I'm not allowed to pick her up**. I'm going to anyway.
T	: What happens?
John	: She's quiet and sleeps.
T	: Go on.
John	: They're **back!** [panicky] I must put her back!
T	: How are you feeling?
John	: My head is sore!! [His first migraine].
T	: What purpose does the pain have?
John	: It reminds me I'm alive.
T	: So it's protecting you. Is there any other purpose?
John	: It's punishing me. Because I picked her up.

Realising he had indeed done the right thing, that it was ridiculous for his parents to have left him with the responsibility of baby-sitting while forbidding him to pick her up, he was able to remove the guilt and ensure a long term cure, not only for his migraine, but for his depression, anxiety and related disorders.

Today, he is fulfilling his true potential - to speak to him is refreshing, he is so alive. He is making it work for himself and his family and deserves every reward.

CHAPTER TWO

Clinical Hypnosis

Minds are like parachutes; they only function when they're open.
Lord Dewar

Just what is hypnosis, really? Let us examine it in a fairly non-scientific way.

A great many people have studied the phenomenon and there is no, repeat no, global and simple definition. This does not surprise me and it should not surprise you the reader either, unless one happens to be wholly scientific in one's approach and demands some unequivocal evidence that can be measured in terms of science.

Science is a most wonderful thing - it has improved our lives to an extent unimaginable just a century ago. Mostly, science has benefited us in a very positive way. We have TV, we have air travel, amazing communication systems, technology in the home - the refrigerator, the microwave oven. We have satellites and have landed a man - several men - on the moon. We have MRI scanners as a commonplace investigation in medical clinics. Scientific method has achieved this and it owes a great deal to Des Cartes some hundreds of years ago and to Isaac Newton. In fact, it is termed 'Cartesian-Newtonian science', the 'reductionist' approach - reducing everything to its most basic components. We do indeed owe a great deal to our forefathers.

The problem is we have lost our way in important endeavours with this obsession for hard science. Everything must be measurable. If one cannot measure it, one cannot publish one's findings and one cannot believe it. It is not a great step to then say "it doesn't exist". Well, there is a star cluster in the Tarantula Nebula known as R136. With the best available ground-based telescopes, it was originally thought that this celestial object was a 'supermassive star'. The advent of the Hubble space telescope allowed a different perspective - far from being the anomaly of a supermassive star, it is now very evident that R136 is a cluster of more than three thousand individual stars! Of course, it is easy to believe this because we can **see** it.

The human mind … any mind, except for an artificial intelligence construct, cannot be measured. One can monitor it by electroencephalography, or EEG. One can do magnetic resonance imagery or MRI scan. One can even do scans that pinpoint where the neuronal activity is taking place in the mind. However, one cannot measure **why** a thought arises, nor even **how**. When, maybe. Where, maybe. But this is measuring **after** the fact. One cannot measure the soul. They - scientists - have tried repeatedly to determine this phenomenon of 'consciousness' … and have failed miserably.

So it is very difficult to give an accurate, global, biophysical definition that will satisfy the scientific diehards. As Gindes stated : *"Few fields of science have suffered as much from the encumbrances of poor definition as Hypnosis."* Hypnosis is perhaps more an art than it is a science.

If I were challenged to give a definition of hypnosis, there are two I could offer, because they are simple. Patricia Honiotes defines it as: *A state of direct or indirect concentration, with or without relaxation, in which a person may accept or reject suggestions, good or bad.* Dr Daniel Zelling's definition is much more succint - *Expectancy and Acceptance.*

However, we can certainly provide a description of the characteristics of hypnosis. By doing this, we can allay much of the fear that is associated with it. The fear of hypnosis is prevalent and warrants some exploration because it is one of the causes of failed or only partially successful therapy.

There are three aspects to this fear. Firstly, there is the influence of the Church, of organised religion – or at least of some of the Western religions. When the Roman Empire embraced Catholicism as the state religion, hypnosis was declared a heresy; it was banned, it was declared evil. This was reconfirmed in Constantinople in the 2nd century. I have no doubt that this was done with good intent, to protect citizens from potential abuse. However, it was Man who did the banning, not God. The ability to enter trance is inherent in all of us. Had God not intended this, I find it most unlikely that He would have provided us with this gift. But, if the religious powers that be say **no** - with the risk of and to the point of damnation - it is a powerful negative influence, and one which grew with time.

There is also the objection, particularly from certain churches, that all hypnosis dabbles in the occult - that it is the work of the devil. Hypnosis can be misused - but so can religion or medicine. The concept of 'possession' is, in my opinion, and more importantly in that of respected academics, an 'introject'. An introjection is the subconscious incorporation into one's personality of the characteristics of another person or inanimate object.

The point is, that particular person chooses to incorporate this idea into himself - it is not enforced by an outside agent. Such a person is found to have a vulnerability in that there is an Identity Problem or a Jurisdictional Problem - both of which will be discussed later. A patient with significant guilt may well incorporate the outside concept of the devil into himself, because that is how he feels about himself - evil; this is so in the patients I have treated - it is to them a fitting self-punishment for their guilt.

Furthermore, I have doubts that 'possession' introjects would ever occur had not our religious history provided the concept in the first place. I believe the more it is publicised from the pulpit or in the media, the more likely we shall see such unnecessary tragedies.

The second aspect of the fear of hypnosis is a fear of confronting the origin of the fear itself - hidden in the subconscious. To the subconscious, this may be perceived as still far too threatening. The reasons why will become apparent later.

The third aspect of fear is the faulty belief that one loses control. This is consequent on another faulty belief that hypnotic trance is a deep sleep in which one is unaware of what is happening, that one does not remember what has occurred - that for all practical purposes, one is in a type of coma or in deep anaesthesia. This is of course, untrue. More to the point is that even in a coma or under anaesthesia, the subconscious mind is **still** functioning and receives information through the senses. The fact that patients are aware of what is happening in the operating theatre has been confirmed by more than one worker. A colleague of mine - one of my teachers, Dr Bernard Levinson - researched this and confirmed the phenomenon in the nineteen fifties!! Of course, his work was quietly ignored by academia.

An article on February 24, 1996 in the daily Johannesburg newspaper, *The Star*, describes two coma patients who recovered from a declared brain dead 'vegetative' state. One patient had suffered the 'bends' in a diving accident and was in a coma for six months. On the day his life support systems were to be switched off, his mother begged for a 'stay of execution'. Just as well - a few days later he awoke to report he had heard every word of the conversations during that time. The other patient was a New York policeman who was in a coma for seven years after a gunshot wound; he remembered with clarity what had occurred during those years.

Clearly, a flat line electroencephalogram does not mean with certainty that a patient is dead. We have to reassess not only the medical management of these patients, but also acknowledge that the brain and spirit are far more resilient than we had thought at a scientific level. There is now research into techniques that will help us to improve accuracy in diagnosing those who may be recoverable.

Essentially, hypnosis is a state of altered consciousness in which many things occur and I will briefly discuss two of them. Firstly, far from being asleep, in trance one is very much more alert and awake compared to our normal wakeful state. One can see, hear, taste, touch and smell better. One can think and remember with greater clarity. Directional sense is greatly enhanced - *The Soul of the Ape* by Eugene Marais discusses this phenomenon in more detail.

Together with this increased alertness there is usually but not always an increased relaxation response. Muscles relax, tensions dissipate, the blood pressure tends to come down, the heart rate reduces, breathing becomes slower and more measured. Endorphins are released in greater quantities – these are morphine-like peptides or chemicals produced by the body which induce a sense of peace and well-being, as well as reducing the perception of pain. The body's ability to combat infection is increased.

One is now relaxed but very alert and still able to think. It follows that one retains the power to choose to accept **or** reject any suggestion that is given. The person who allows the trance to occur in the first place is the patient! To be more accurate, the patient's subconscious mind. One puts oneself in trance, not the therapist - he or she acts only as a guide, as a catalyst.

The subconscious mind is **very** powerful - more so than the conscious mind: emotion holds sway over logic. The single duty and goal of the subconscious is the **survival** of that individual. Should any threat be perceived - whether it be financial, physical, emotional, intellectual or spiritual, the subconscious is **compelled** to act in some appropriate way to ensure the survival of that person. If the act of entering trance is perceived as threatening, it will not occur. In simple terms, **the patient has the control** - always. One cannot be made to do in trance anything one would not do **out** of trance. It is a question of self-trust, nothing more. However, one can be tricked into hypnosis, even though consciously one does not want to go into trance. For this reason, if no other, one is advised to avoid situations with non-professionals.

In terms of not doing things in trance that are against one's moral principles, as I tell my patients, "suppose you are now in a deep trance and I suggest that you take off all your clothes, run around the block and then come back and sit down. If you think 'that's OK, that'll be fun', you might well do it. However, if you think 'no way, that is absolutely against my principles' you will not carry out the suggestion. It is much more likely that you will come out of trance, aim a blow at me and head for the nearest attorney. The next time I see you will be in court - and no doubt about it, at the Health Professions Council too!"

We are aware that the non-dominant half of the brain has to do with the subconscious. Most people believe that the dominant or thinking, logical side is switched off under hypnosis. This is simply not true. One retains the ability to think, to way up the pros and cons of a situation - more so than usual, normally. It is rather that the logical brain parks on the side of the road in neutral, to observe. It will not interfere unless called upon to do so in the presence of some threat.

Stage hypnotists - and I have little respect for some of their behaviour - who claim, when they have a group of people on the stage in trance, that they are in control of the group have a problem. Either they lack knowledge or, what is worse, they may have a need to be in control. It is not a situation I would like any member of my family to be in. People on the stage who do those silly, frivolous things do so only because they are not threatened by the suggestions given to them. Far more dangerous is the situation where a person's subconscious is bent on self-destruction ... for whatever reason. The stage hypnotist has no idea of this and may provide suggestions which are potentially devastating. For the most part though, I would hazard a guess that many of these people **like** to be up there on the stage - it lends a sense of importance… it boosts the ego. Alternatively they may feel more threatened by being labelled as cowards for refusing to go up on stage. If so, the lesser threat will be followed and their hypnotisability increased - much to the delight of the stage hypnotist, who appears to be a really powerful personality, which he is not. If the hypnotist suggests that nothing will be remembered after the trance state, again the subconscious may choose to accept or reject this suggestion - so the patient may not **consciously** recall the events on the stage. Yet the subconscious mind can, and does recall, which is why we are able to reverse any damage incurred as a result of stage hypnosis. And such problems can and do occur. Non-professional hypnosis will be discussed in more detail later.

This fear of losing control leads to other fears, for example: "If I go into this hypnotic trance, is there a chance I will never come out of it?" Again, the answer is no, one will always wake up, even if not given the suggestion to do so. If the therapist should suddenly die from a heart attack, one will immediately know something is wrong - one would spontaneously wake up. If the therapist should quietly walk out, one would know. If one were enjoying the peacefulness, one might elect to remain in trance. However, if one knew that one had an appointment elsewhere in half an hour, one would similarly re-alert oneself.

A further fear is that deep and dark secrets will be told by the patient. This is simply not true ... and sometimes I wish it were so, because it may be a deep and dark secret that is responsible for the presenting symptom! If I were indeed in control, I would be able to help each and every patient resolve forever all their problems. Clearly this is not the case. There is no power that I have that can elicit something the patient does not want to part with. A hopeful woman called me one day with a problem. One of their company's trucks had been hijacked and they suspected that the driver was involved. She wanted me to find out if this was so. I had to answer her: "If you want to pay me for my time, that's fine. But if he wishes to, he will lie to me like a cheap watch." There was a stunned disbelieving silence on the other end of the telephone, but it is true. If a patient is awake and I'm threatening him - possibly eliciting information that will send him to jail - it is unlikely he will tell me the truth!

As I hinted at earlier, hypnotic trance is a God-given ability we all possess. It is a **natural** phenomenon - we all experience trance at least twice a day. That period of time between wakefulness and sleep is a state of hypnosis. It may last only some seconds if one is really tired. At other times it may last many minutes. My elder brother is blessed with this ability - he says he experiences it every night for ten or more minutes. Similarly, that period of time when one wakes up, before full alertness, is a state of hypnosis. Physiologically it is a state of *alpha rhythm* – rather midway between normal sleep and full wakefulness and is no different to yoga or other meditation.

There are many other examples - daydreaming or fantasising are classic examples. One can sit in a classroom or at work and, in the mind's eye, find oneself transported to the beach, or into the arms of one's boyfriend. Physically one is in class, but in one's mind one is miles away ... at least until rapped on the back of the hand by the teacher, jerking one back to reality. Never mind, at least in retrospect painful knuckles demonstrate a talent for self-hypnosis.

Another common experience is arriving home to realise that one does not quite remember turning those last three or four corners. Whatever happened? How did one get there? Usually in this situation one has been focussing consciously on some train of thought while the subconscious mind has taken all the necessary steps to bring one home - quite safely, I might add. Should some emergency have arisen, for example a dog or a child running across the road, there would still be an automatic survival intervention.

The unnoticed passage of time while driving on a long journey or while engrossed in a really good novel are other examples. A trick I used unknowingly, while at university, was to play music tapes or records while studying. My conscious mind initially tuned in to the music but after a while I realised that while working away diligently the tape had stopped without my noticing. The music had provided the distraction for my conscious ... my subconscious focussed on the work.

When I saw the first Rambo movie, the rest of the audience might as well have been on the planet Mars - I was **in** that film! I was Stallone's shadow man, listening for every sound, watching for any subtle change around me ... in the film! My surroundings had become unimportant - my attention was on the storyline, the adventure.

So the fact is that we have all experienced trance. In a therapeutic situation we utilise this to achieve some sort of positive result. For example, I am sometimes consulted by students suffering from examination anxiety. These poor souls, many of them far more clever than I am, have done all the work. They know their stuff. But, on entering the examination hall panic takes over, quite literally. Some of them have a genuine panic attack, with over-breathing or hyperventilation, palpitations, dizziness - the whole catastrophe, including the loss of the ability to think calmly and rationally ... or to remember anything! In analysis, we find that most of them have had a previous life-threatening experience - most commonly the birth experience.

It is not very difficult to take them back to that first panic situation, to let them realise the danger is over and that an examination provides no real threat. They are able to relate their panic attack to the life or death situation of the birth experience - the reason for all hyperventilation. Bingo, 'exam nerves' disappear. What's more, having also realised that there is nothing wrong with their memory it is again a relatively simple matter to enhance recall of what they have studied. Obviously, their marks improve - by as much as ten percent!

Hypnosis, then, involves a narrowing of a focus of attention with distraction from the immediate environment. A part of the subconscious will always remain aware of the immediate surroundings and provide any necessary intervention in an emergency. This part of the mind was called the 'hidden observer' by Dr Watkins. In this state of trance, suggestions may be given to the patient - and it is important to realise that these suggestions may be accepted **or** rejected by the mind. Again, this demonstrates the control the patient retains.

Research shows that between ten and fifteen percent of the population have a remarkably good talent for hypnosis - so much so that they can totally eliminate pain, stop bleeding and so on, which is very useful in surgery! It is possible for these fortunate people to undergo major surgery with no chemical anaesthetic at all, just hypno-anaesthesia. This is the group whom stage hypnotists like to call up onto the platform - it's very easy to work with them and the hypnotist appears to be some kind of genius, which he is not. Clever and manipulative he certainly is. A showman - an entertainer, yes. But a genius? Not really.

Another seventy percent of people are able to readily enter into trance. The remainder have difficulty going into trance in a formal situation, not because they cannot - we all are in trance twice a day at least - but because of fear. This fear may be a conscious one: if one does not consciously trust the hypnotist, no trance will happen. It may also be a subconscious fear. So even if a person is desperate for help, if his subconscious says "no", it is "**no**". I have had five patients who could not achieve even the lightest of trances. It is of interest that two of them were born behind the then Iron Curtain in East Germany. As children they were repeatedly given the suggestion to trust no-one, for fear of risking the lives of the whole family. Such a block is difficult indeed to remove.

By and large, there are only two ways in which a patient can be assisted in hypnosis. One is by suggestion - direct or indirect. Let me explain this a little more. I can give a direct suggestion to a person with anxiety that he will become progressively more relaxed not only in the trance, but also afterwards - during his normal waking hours. An indirect suggestion achieves the same result. Instead of simply saying, "You will feel more relaxed", I can tell him a story that suggests the same thing; or utilise some type of metaphor. As the subconscious has a leaning towards picture stories, such suggestions implied by the metaphor may have great power in assisting us towards the goal.

The other method is by analysis, in which the source of any particular symptom is searched for, understood and eliminated. This takes more time, but is certainly more successful and usually achieves much longer lasting relief, usually permanent. There are different methods of analysis. Those most commonly used are Medical Hypnoanalysis, Ego State Therapy and Traditional Hypnoanalysis. Anaylsis in trance is not a new idea at all - Breuer first recognised (at least in the Western world) in 1880 that repressed trauma may be the cause of a symptom and the emphasis of therapeutic hypnosis began to change from direct suggestion to symptom removal.

Elsewhere, many cultures have utilised and continue to utilise hypnosis in their own way. More primitive cultures used the rhythm of drums, for example, to induce a trance state, others make use of certain naturally occurring toxins including hallucinogens - substances which alter one's psyche. Fakirs (Muslim or Hindu religious mendicants) have for thousands of years used hypnosis, as have shamans and many others such as the Persian Magi, or priestly caste. The Egyptians and ancient Greeks had 'sleep temples' - the Temple of Aesculapius is an example. The Romans also made use of hypnosis.

Jewish readers may now realise that 'davening' is an induction of hypnotic trance - the purpose of which is to facilitate a focussed state of mind and to be more easily in touch with the Divine. Davening, to those Gentiles who hopefully are also reading this book, is a rhythmic swaying of the body to and fro, while praying. In fact, hypnosis was widely used and accepted until the intervention of orthodox Christian religion. In the Western world, hypnosis took an unfortunate 'dive', from which it is only now slowly starting to recover.

At this time we need to understand that hypnosis is not a treatment in itself, although the relaxation it brings is an advantage and may have therapeutic benefits. Rather, hypnotic trance is the medium in which a patient is treated. So, one may use behavioural therapy, cognitive therapy, sex therapy or any number of other therapies **in** trance. Which type is used will depend on the individual therapist's training and preference. It will also depend on the patient's needs. It is also important to understand that hypnosis is not the be-all and end-all of treatments - far from it! It is not a miracle cure-all and should not detract in any way from any needed conventional medical or psychological treatment. It is a complementary tool that can and does allow conventional medicine and psychology to be more coherent and effective ... and often much more rapidly.

A number of phenomena occur in hypnotic trance which would be interesting to explore.

Amnesia can be induced by suggestion. A subject can be told that there is no number six, and then asked to count his fingers. This is a classic stage trick which causes much mirth in the audience, while creating confusion and embarrassment in the subject – and is therefore to be deplored. Because when he counts his fingers, he misses out 'six' and is left with a spare finger or thumb on reaching 'ten'. This is not a pleasant experience - it is disconcerting and confusing and may result in a great deal of anxiety.

Regression is a characteristic of hypnosis. A subject can go back to a previous time in his life to re-experience his perceptions. So if a patient's subconscious gives the therapist permission, he can be taken back to his third birthday and will quite happily relate what presents he received, the type of cake and what it tasted like, who was there and so on. Regression can occur by suggestion and guidance ... it can also occur spontaneously.

The danger here is that such a regression may recall unwelcome experiences and create a crisis. In untrained hands, the consequences may be serious for this person, and even precipitate a psychosis. This is another reason for the discouragement of non-professional or lay hypnotists who seem to be unaware of the pyschological damage they can cause. These individuals, with no formal training in psychology or medicine, attend a course for a couple of weekends and are presented with a certificate proclaiming them to be hypnotists, which implies that they are now qualified to treat medical and psychological ills. Some even complete a three or four week course to become 'master hypnotists'. Well, by their own standards they may be qualified.

Four weeks to master status! It takes seven **years,** up to eight in the new South Africa, to qualify as a general practitioner; a psychologist studies for almost as long. Only post-graduate medical students are trained in hypnosis and its advanced techniques. Some lay hypnotists are to my mind potentially even more dangerous than stage hypnotists. To reach the highest qualification in the South African Society of Clinical Hypnosis requires diligent work and study for a minimum of five years at post-graduate level, under peer review and after appropriate examinations.

Another favourite and very common trick of the stage hypnotist is the use of the phenomenon of 'post-hypnotic suggestion'. "When you wake up you will believe you are Elvis Presley and sing Jailhouse Rock." The audience collapses laughing at the spectacle, the subject is embarrassed. Some people are outraged. Is this abuse? I believe it is open to abuse. I once watched a British TV program on hypnosis, where the stage hypnotist suggested to a young female subject that he was her favourite male film star. Not only did he neglect to reverse this suggestion, he announced to the audience that this was "one of the perks of the job"!! Had that hypnotist been a member of the South African Society of Clinical Hypnosis, I can tell you categorically that our recommendation to the Health Professions Council would be to revoke his licence to practise. Many professionals - and I use the word in its strictest sense - have seen negative results of lay or stage hypnotherapy. There is literature on the subject.

The stage hypnotist does not take much of a history, before the show. With luck, and depending on the individual, he may refuse to hypnotise anyone being treated for an emotional disorder or one who is taking 'recreational' drugs, which is eminently sensible. However, he knows nothing else about that person. Imagine a person who has had a near drowning in the sea at the age of two and who is given the suggestion to imagine himself wading in the sea ... there is every possibility that the subconscious will immediately relive this old fear, resulting in a panic attack on the stage, or later. There is no trained professional in this country who is not aware of the need to take a proper history - forewarned is forearmed, and in therapy this type of circumstance is exactly what the professional is seeking as a cause of the patient's problem. I require a minimum of one hour to take a history from a patient - a stage hypnotist takes perhaps one or two minutes.

There is a belief among stage hypnotists that they do not do age regression on the stage - this is not true. I will allow that they may not do so deliberately, but nevertheless age regression commonly occurs in stage hypnosis - spontaneously! People who experience nausea, vomiting, headaches and so on with or after stage hypnosis **have** experienced regression to an earlier time of threat associated with these symptoms. They are abreacting, that is reliving uncomfortable and distressing memories, but the stage or lay hypnotist may not realise this fact. Is this evidence of irresponsibility, or ignorance? I do not allow any patient of mine who comes out of trance with these or similar symptoms to go home until we have re-induced hypnosis and resolved the symptom, or at least modified it until such time as we do resolve it. Failure to do this would amount to professional neglect. The statement that these symptoms are merely side effects of stage hypnosis is misleading. It is misinformation, whether deliberate or through ignorance, and it is simply not true. There is a growing body of professional literature which disputes this belief. Furthermore, stage hypnotists do not fall under any statutory body of control. Whilst anybody can induce hypnosis (it's not difficult), **not** everybody can safely and constructively utilise it for others in a clinical setting. I have no doubt this is one of the major reasons the Church banned hypnosis nearly two thousand years ago.

The belief that stage hypnosis does not cause embarrassment to the individual is also largely untrue. We have all laughed at jokes in which someone was a 'fall-guy'. All humour is based on something unfortunate. On the stage, I submit, it is the hypnotised individual who is unfortunate. While it is the subconscious which ultimately chooses to go into trance, subjects can be tricked into it. Enough said on this subject.

Dissociation is another phenomenon which is useful. For example, it can be suggested to a patient with a terminal and painful disease to become 'separated' or 'switched off' from his pain-wracked body. It can be suggested that he is enjoying a movie in another room, while leaving his pain in the bedroom.

Time distortion occurs naturally in trance - an hour's session may be perceived by the subject as fifteen minutes. In fact a good subject can be trained to compress time to such a degree that he can review his entire matric science syllabus in half an hour. I have seen a subject listen to his complete (and extensive) jazz collection in five minutes! When I attended a concert by the late jazz pianist Dave Brubeck I perceived the 2 and a half hour concert had lasted only twenty minutes!

Pain control and anaesthesia can be achieved by a patient with varying degrees of success. As mentioned above, about ten percent of people have a talent for hypnosis so developed that they can undergo surgery without any chemical anaesthetic agent. Most people can achieve a dramatic reduction of pain. Imagine painless childbirth - wonderful! Just as wonderful as pain-free dentistry! There are patients who fall into the so-called ten percent of poor hypnotic ability, who with the development of trust in themselves, can and do achieve total pain control, at will.

The physiology of the body may be altered in hypnosis. The subconscious controls all the automatic functions of the body such as blood pressure, heart rate, breathing, bleeding and so on and this can be utilised clinically.

In January 1996 the Johannesburg **Sunday Times** newspaper published a story of a crocodile attack in which four friends came to the rescue of the victim. They battled the croc and victim to the rocky bank but could not lift him and his attacker out of the water. Three of them got out as quickly as possible to find some means of saving him, leaving a young man weighing just 65 kg as the only link to his friend's survival. He held on desperately, trying to buy time for the others to come with help. The croc however, began to pull the victim down again. At that moment he knew that if he did not do something, his friend would disappear forever. From a sitting position he lifted both his 85 kg friend and a 168 kg crocodile out of the water onto his lap in a superhuman effort! Superhuman? The absolute **need**? Divine intervention? Whatever the answer, there is clearly an immense energy and power latent in a human being. I have no doubt that the hero was in trance - he was totally focussed on the survival situation, He **knew** what had to be done ... and simply did it. This brave young man provides an example of the love inherent in Man. He risked his own life for another.

The immune system can be enhanced under hypnosis, enabling a patient to combat disease. There are many anecdotal and published accounts of the ability of a person to utilise this inner strength in many varied diseases. Our immune status' efficiency is directly related to the state of our spirit. A renowned doctor from Florida, USA Dr Simonton, who works with cancer patients, found that he "couldn't get patients with advanced cancer to comply with treatment in a positive way. They saw no reason to involve themselves, **because they had no confidence in their ability to get well**" (my emphasis). In medical hypnoanalysis we call this lack of hope, this acceptance of death, the Walking Zombie Syndrome. Once the mind has accepted death emotionally and spiritually, the physical body is not far behind. It is often seen that when a spouse dies, especially after many years of marriage, the other follows within months. They have no more purpose in life ... and they simply die. In other words, there is much still to be achieved in therapy at a far deeper level than the purely physical.

Dr Ornish, of California USA, showed that coronary artery disease can be stabilised and cholesterol levels lowered using normal dietary measures and imagery techniques. Dr Sheinman reported a case of scleroderma with kidney failure. A patient who would not have had more than a couple of years, if that, to live was apparently healed with guided imagery in trance. Using analytical hypnosis techniques I have patients with Lupus Erythematosus, ulcerative colitis and Crohn's disease who have turned their backs on their disease and chosen to live.

Dr Dabney Ewin, an American surgeon, demonstrated the effectiveness of hypnosis in serious third-degree burns, to the extent of avoiding skin grafts which would otherwise have been imperative.

Dr Daniel Zelling described a case of multiple sclerosis which was resolved with medical hypnoanalysis. I had a patient with AIDS whom we were treating for an anxiety issue spontaneously raise her CD-4 count from 200 to 400 as her anxiety resolved.

A few years ago I 'popped' two lumbar discs, confirmed on MRI scanning, resulting in extreme pain and loss of function – could hardly walk. Surgery had to be delayed for ten days as I was taking anti-coagulants. Using hypnotic imagery I saw those two discs as grapes shrinking down to small raisins and in four days I was pain free and fully mobile – even swinging my golf clubs. I avoided major surgery.

Clearly, each individual has a vast potential to promote and maintain his or her own health. It is a scandal that this gift is not utilised. More time and money are spent on our motor cars than on our own wellbeing. Cars are serviced regularly, but our bodies and minds are often neglected. It would take perhaps a mere five or ten minutes, twice a day, to change all this. And there is always time.

To harness this power, we must begin to look at our inner spiritual selves. We need to add to our scientific knowledge so that the very essence of life may be maximised. Some years ago I wrote a couple of articles to encourage that exploration in this country.

The classic, simplistic scientific approach is to question why, how, what, where and when - and then to apply scientific method to prove or disprove an assumption or theory. Since Des Cartes, all our endeavours have followed this route and to step off the highway was to invite being ostracised - at least from the scientific community. Many academics promote this amputation, and I suspect that one reason they do so is because they may feel threatened. Whenever a challenge is issued, it is human nature to retaliate - survival is imperative. This is what our subconscious minds are striving for, even if it makes no intellectual sense. Of course, just as many are concerned that reasonable procedures should be followed for the good of the public, ultimately for the good of humanity. This is their particular reason for being critical - and rightly so.

The strange thing is, actually the tragedy is, that they are usually unwilling to co-operate in 'reasonable' trials. I once asked the head of a Department of Rheumatology, after suitable discussion, whether his department would not design, manage and control a trial in the use of Medical Hypnoanalysis for rheumatoid arthritis. The response was guarded. My requested written proposal did not even elicit a response. I had been relegated to the 'crazy fringe' and for them it was not worth the risk of international and/or academic ridicule. The same is true in the USA and elsewhere - my colleagues there and in the United Kingdom report the same armoured door slamming in their faces. Science is not just 'king', it is everything.

Ironically, some doubt has begun to be cast on the holy grail of 'scientific method' - for example (and there are many others) St Clair Gibson from Cape Town has the opinion that random double-blind trials have become so rigidly controlled that it is now problematic to draw conclusions. The question is raised whether these research protocols can be applied to the general population, the reason being that every possible variable is kept the same for each person in the trial. However, as each person has his or her own individual physiological response to certain conditions, it really is impossible to draw absolute conclusions. I would add that each person has his or her own individual learned subconscious responses to certain conditions! What St Clair Gibson did not state, but I'm sure implied, is that a person's emotional response may vary, influencing the physiology and hence the result. Many trials represent an artificially constructed environment. If only **one** person in a trial has a beneficial result with placebo (a substance with no physiological effect) then one simply has to question the validity of any result.

Things are not what they seem, and even previously rigidly adhered-to laws of physics are showing cracks. At the University of California, Berkeley, researchers led by Raymond Chiao examined the speed of light. Among the experiments they carried out was one in which a photon beam was directed through a curved multi-layered mirror. The majority of the photons were reflected, as expected. What was astounding was that the photons that made it through arrived at the sensor behind the mirror some **seventy** percent **earlier** than expected!

Apparently, the speed of light is **not** absolute. Perhaps a photon is not an indivisible entity.

If this is so, Einstein's E=MC to the second power is not valid under the conditions of the Big Bang and a black hole - and all of physics must then be questioned. What scientific validity does a double-blind trial hold if the speed of light can be shown to be 306000 miles rather than 180000 miles per second? We're in trouble. With our present level of scientific knowledge, we cannot even account for at least forty percent of the mass in this universe! Although we have now identified the Higgs boson it is found to be of a mass trillions of times less than it's supposed to be. What is truth, then? What really does the universe represent, what do we represent? As Dr Dan Zelling pointed out, "it is not so much that you believe it when you see it - you see it when you believe it!"

In financial terms, hypnosis may be far more cost-effective for many people. A 1990's report in a medical journal described a patient who was unsuccessfully treated by a psychiatrist, until rescued by another! This patient was taking **ten** different drugs, of which nine were psychoactive, at a cost of R1400 a month at that time. The patient had been treated for four years until admitted to hospital for six weeks for detoxification and intensive psychotherapy. The cost of hospitalisation at that time was R300 per day. The patient was discharged on a rational dose of just one antidepressant. When one adds up all the expenses, including that of consultations by psychiatrists and psychologists, one is looking at an astronomical sum close to R90,000! This excludes the loss of earnings. This patient might have been successfully treated by a hypnotherapist at a fraction of the cost.

Research in Switzerland indicates that the costs of managing Multiple Sclerosis amounts to 50,000 Swiss Francs a year. Dr Daniel Zelling published a paper describing a patient who cured himself from this disease at a cost far, far less than that.

Stephen Hawking, in his book **'A Brief History of Time',** says "the history of science has been the gradual realisation that events do not happen in an arbitrary manner, but that they reflect a certain underlying order, which may or may not be divinely inspired." He continues later: "the real test is whether predictions agree with observation." If this

is so, "we could be reasonably confident that the predictions are the right ones." Repeatability is a cornerstone of scientific method. Medical Hypnoanalysis certainly has achieved that consistency over more than sixty years and its predictions should now, to my thinking, be considered for acceptance by the wider community of the healing sciences.

CHAPTER THREE

Of Mind, Body and Spirit

That is the essence of science: ask an impertinent question and you are on the way to a pertinent answer.
       J. Bronowski; The Ascent of Man, 1973.

He uses statistics as a drunken man uses lamp-posts - for support rather than illumination.
       Andrew Lang; quoted by
    A.L. Mackay in Harvest of a Quiet Eye.

I can already feel the hackles rising. I can imagine, even hear pen being applied to paper or fingers to keyboard in an indignant response. It's OK. Figuratively speaking, I have broad shoulders. I have even made such responses myself in my own days of blind or blinkered belief in the scientific method. Nor do I reject the scientific principles I was taught. We must after all manage our problems in the real world - we must be realistic. But now I know more of the truth - not anywhere near all truth of course, but more. There is a growing body of evidence that many diseases - both physical and psychological - have a source that is not primarily genetic, inherited or congenital, ie not primarily a physiological process. This evidence is undeniable and irresistible. In time I trust there will be reasonable co-operation between the two schools of thought because the reason for our work, on both sides of and straddling the fence, is for the benefit of our fellow human beings. That is the goal… that is the essence of the Hippocratic Oath. That is the human spirit.

  The divergence arises because whilst one can measure physical occurrences, one cannot measure emotion. One cannot measure the human spirit. Those who say "Nonsense, of course we can!" are misled. What we measure in the human body are the **physical manifestations** of emotion. Not **the** emotion. We are measuring the effect of adrenalin on the pulse rate or blood pressure. We are measuring the biochemical responses of cortisone and other chemicals to stress. We are **not** measuring feelings or even thoughts - and that certainly includes electroencephalography or SPECT scans. Consider the following diagram, which seeks to combine our scientific knowledge of human suffering in one model:

The Newtonian-Einsteinan-Quantum Theory Diagram of Disease

The outer circle represents the scientific theory, the middle circle the symptom of the patient and the inner circle the disease process or pathological mechanism. The patient arrives in the doctor's rooms and declares "I have a sore throat." The doctor examines the patient and finds a streptococcal throat infection. Good - we have some objectivity from the Newtonian scientific perspective.

The patient goes on to add "You know, doctor, I felt rotten for weeks before the sore throat began." Very well, here is a subjective observation of stress which we can associate with Einstein's Theory of Relativity. Indeed, if we examine the patient's immune response, we might find it wanting - why he got the infection in the first place.

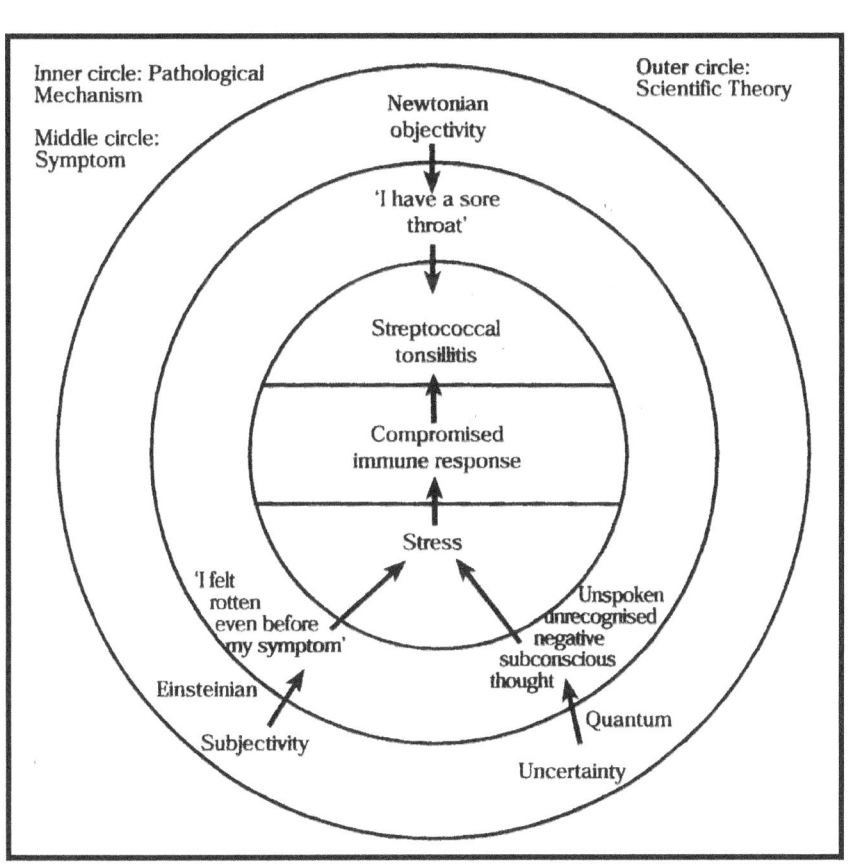

However, he also has a negative subconscious thought not recognised even by himself which also negatively affects his immune response: this represents Heisenberg's Uncertainty Principle in Quantum Mechanics. This, in brief, states that we cannot know the exact position of an atom's electron as well as its energy **at the same time.** What do you know even the physicists are at a loss: nothing is exact! If physics breaks down at sub-nuclear levels, are not Newtonian and Einsteinian theories again cast in some doubt?

The Hubble telescope has added to our confusion. It provides the most accurate measurements of the age of the universe to date. Whereas previously the age of the universe was estimated at fifteen or more billion years, now it has been determined to be around 13.82 billion years. Yet with our best estimation, the oldest stars are more than fourteen billion years old! Contradictions.

What **do** we know, really? This confusion is the reason for the physicist's goal in trying to find **one** Grand Unification Theory that **will** make sense, and will probably be achieved by current and future work in Multidimensional Superstring Theory and Chaos Theory and a true understanding of Gravity, dark energy and dark matter. Gravitational waves have only recently been discovered. The theoretical physicist Erik Verlinde describes a new theory of gravity as an emergent phenomenon which is possibly derived from the infinitely small building blocks that constitute the universe's existence. In November 2016 he said "gravity emerges from fundamental bits of information stored in the very structure of spacetime". He continues by saying if this is so that 'dark matter' is not required to explain what's happening in galaxies and has evidence that this new concept agrees with observations.

In any event, there may be a great deal going on behind this apparently straightforward throat infection.

By the very nature of our Western culture, we have been taught and channelled into a narrow focus of Newtonian values. This focus often falsely implies that the 'what' of a disease also explains the 'why'. More experienced and perhaps wiser members of the healing professions, mostly psychiatrists and psychologists, venture into the Einsteinian Subjectivity theory. However, very few perceive the Quantum

Uncertainty of Subconscious influence. One of my teachers even denied that such a thing as the subconscious exists! "A memory bank, that's all." This same academic once concluded in exasperation at a clinical meeting: "Alright! There are some people who were born depressed and will remain so forever. There is nothing we can do for them!" He was both right and wrong: right because the majority of depressed people are indeed born depressed. However, many workers in the USA, in South Africa and Australia now find the reason for this is that they had **already** accepted their own death, or that life was no longer worth living, while still in the womb, or while **being** born. He was wrong because we **can** do much to correct this faulty belief.

Still fewer healers consider the spiritual self and its influence on health.

With this kind of teaching, many doctors are in trouble. They have a vague awareness of the influence of the spirit and mind, nod their heads sagely but are uncertain as to how to approach these matters, or what to do. It is far easier to ignore them. "It's not my responsibility. My waiting room is too full to warrant such discussions with my patients." And of course they are right - the average doctor has little or no training in these matters and they are too time-consuming. The total psychology course I attended as an undergraduate consisted of just eight one-hour lectures in the fourth year of study. However, referral to another doctor or psychologist who does have the time and expertise will ultimately **reduce** both the costs and duration of the illness in many cases - a fact which medical insurers have yet to realise!

Many doctors have enough to worry about - and yes, doctors **do** worry about their patients - never doubt that. They are simply trying to get through the day in a minefield of pathological biochemistry which is mushrooming daily while trying to maintain human contact. Thus it becomes easier and easier to prescribe, rather than to get involved with poorly understood issues. For most patients, this is fine. The majority will improve or 'cope' on medication in a far more comfortable manner. However, when the medication is discontinued, the next time a stressor comes along they are likely to relapse. Not surprisingly, successive crises tend to result in more serious symptoms.

One should never be satisfied with 'coping'. I believe one can do much better if motivated and shown the way. The word 'cope' in this context has its roots in the garment a priest wears over his street clothes - his cope – the robe - **hides** them. By the time they see me or my colleagues most patients are tired of hiding. They may be scared, yes, but they want to break out and be free. They want to **live** rather than continue to obscure themselves.

Healing does not rest solely on the block of polished granite which Westernised medicine believes it is. There are also the cornerstones of mind and spiritual self. To ignore any of the three - body, mind or spirit - is to invite incomplete healing. I believe that in orthodox medicine generally the *status quo* of the patient is merely maintained, postponing matters until the next crisis.

Every doctor has certain patients who make his waiting room a 'second lounge.' There is even a term for them: 'heartsink' patients. What a negative approach! If the doctor believes he cannot help them what chance has the patient? By their very behaviour these people are saying out loud **'I have pain!'** - pain in his or her soul. As the remarkable Milton Erickson pointed out, that pain needs to be recognised and it may be very, very difficult to do so at a conscious level, because the patient himself is not aware of it! It is in his subconscious ... and the subconscious is not generally available to logical thought processes.

As I have mentioned, I have yet to see a patient with an overactive thyroid gland - thyrotoxicosis - who did not have a preceding history of significant anxiety, fear or guilt. Usually one can pin-point what precipitated the condition a year or two beforehand. The same can be said for many cases of high blood pressure, recurrent ovarian cysts, or migraine. It is my belief that the group of diseases such as rheumatoid arthritis, lupus and scleroderma – the auto-immune diseases - are the physical manifestations of subconscious pain related to anxiety, fear and guilt. It is not by chance that these three ogres are called the '**un**holy trinity'. We can add Toxic Shame to the list and call them the 'Four Horsemen of the Apocalypse'! Questioning colleagues regarding their experience in patients with coronary artery disease, breast cysts, eczema, cancer, etc, one hears figures of up to eighty percent of patients whose history and manner indicated pre-existing psychological problems. I once privately predicted a very anxious patient's thyrotoxicosis after her husband abandoned her for another woman. She proved me correct six months later.

We know that stress may severely compromise the immune system - the body's ability to fight infection with antibodies, white cells and so on. We also know that hypnotic trance and the use of simple imagery can reverse this situation - sometimes dramatically. I am aware of two cases in this country in which relaxation, imagery and positive suggestion in trance have reversed chronic osteomyelitis, which is a chronic infection of bone. One case involved a young boy who was scheduled for radical surgery to remove his infected heel bone. Direct suggestion in hypnosis resulted in the complete resolution of the infection - and there are x-rays to confirm this. I similarly treated a patient with chronic osteomyelitis of the tibia - the main bone of the lower leg. Within twenty-four hours, sinuses in his leg which had produced pus daily for nearly two years were dry. Two more sessions and they had closed. This patient also avoided radical surgery. I saw him socially two years later - he had had no further problems. He still owes me the fees for his treatment, of course, but that is another story!

My own experience of migraine patients reveals the eradication of, and continued freedom from, migraine in the majority of cases. Such patients very often open their history with this statement: "I **suffer** from migraine." As suffering is invariably associated with punishment, there is likely to have been an earlier event involving guilt. We could go on and on - the point I am making is: something else is happening somewhere inside the patient, other than the presenting symptom and if we can identify it, ask the appropriate questions as to why, what, how and when, we may be able to resolve a great deal of suffering.

Where does it all begin? Well, that varies from person to person. One problem is the continued avoidance of recognising the ability of the unborn baby to react to both negative and positive experiences in its limited environment.

In 1993, the respected *British Medical Journal* recognised in an editorial that the emotional and cognitive development of an infant may be compromised by maternal depression. The authors refer to no less than twenty-nine papers, all of which are objective in a Newtonian sense. Dr Geraldine Dawson and her colleagues at Washington University have found that the EEG pattern in infants of depressed mothers is reduced in activity in the infants' left frontal lobes.

However, I have two comments. Firstly, the unfortunate mother is 'blamed'. No mention is made either of the influence of the father, or of others such as the grandparents. The danger here is that an impression is given of sole maternal responsibility. This is unfair and adds an extra burden of guilt to the mother. One should bear in mind too that we are dealing primarily with the perceptions of the baby - the mother may be entirely innocent, while the conditions promote problems for the baby. Secondly, the objectivity is limited to postnatal studies, ie only after the birth of the baby - as if a child develops feelings and reactions only after being born. This is an incorrect supposition and ignores the fact that a foetus is just as influenced by its perceptions of events while still in the womb.

Any mother will confirm that their babies react to external influences. If she gets a fright or moves suddenly, or father beats her or arrives home drunk, the baby often mirrors her responses with its own movements. Playing soothing music has a calming effect on the baby. Scientific studies have confirmed all this with EEGs of the fetus. A great deal of evidence exists to show the baby's reaction yet we continue to act as if the baby is as dead as a doornail. Professor Dominick Purpura, past editor of the *Brain Research Journal*, put the start of awareness of the fetus at between twenty-eight and thirty two-weeks, when the brain's neural circuits are as advanced as a new-born's. This is the pure scientific viewpoint. Yet every therapist who does regression to the prenatal period of life consistently has patients who abreact experiences which have occurred much, much earlier ... even prior to the time the mother is aware of the pregnancy. I can understand the necessary conservatism of science in these contentious issues. However, they are not contentious to me, my colleagues, nor to the patients I have treated. There is no doubt in my own mind of the existence of a spiritual and emotional awareness of the baby in the first trimester - within the first thirteen weeks of pregnancy.

I attended the 12th International Congress of Hypnosis and listened to an inexperienced American therapist report in a workshop discussion that she had had a patient who spontaneously regressed to some time which she "could only say was in the womb." She was not an analytical hypnotherapist and was quite terrified by the experience. Indeed, what she had to say was sceptically received by the participants in the discussion. I came to her rescue because I have no doubt that her patient **did** regress to that time.

Stott, Sameroff, Coppolino, Huttunen and Niskanen have reviewed pregnancy, the mother and other factors and cautiously theorise that psychological disturbance, ill health, developmental lag, and behaviour disturbance in the child may follow maternal stresses in pregnancy.

Long experience by medical hypnoanalysts reveals consistent findings - findings which can be, and have been, verified by interviewing the patient's mother. Indeed, prenatal regression is an essential part of any analysis. The conclusion to be drawn is that the child is affected not only at an emotional level, but also at spiritual and behavioural levels, long before birth - as we shall see in the case discussions. The baby **can** think ... but its ability to think with logic is very limited, and is mostly related to survival.

Returning to our diagram ... how does the body respond to a thought? There is now an upsurge in interest in what is called the 'Mind-Body Connection'. Let us explore this with another diagram:

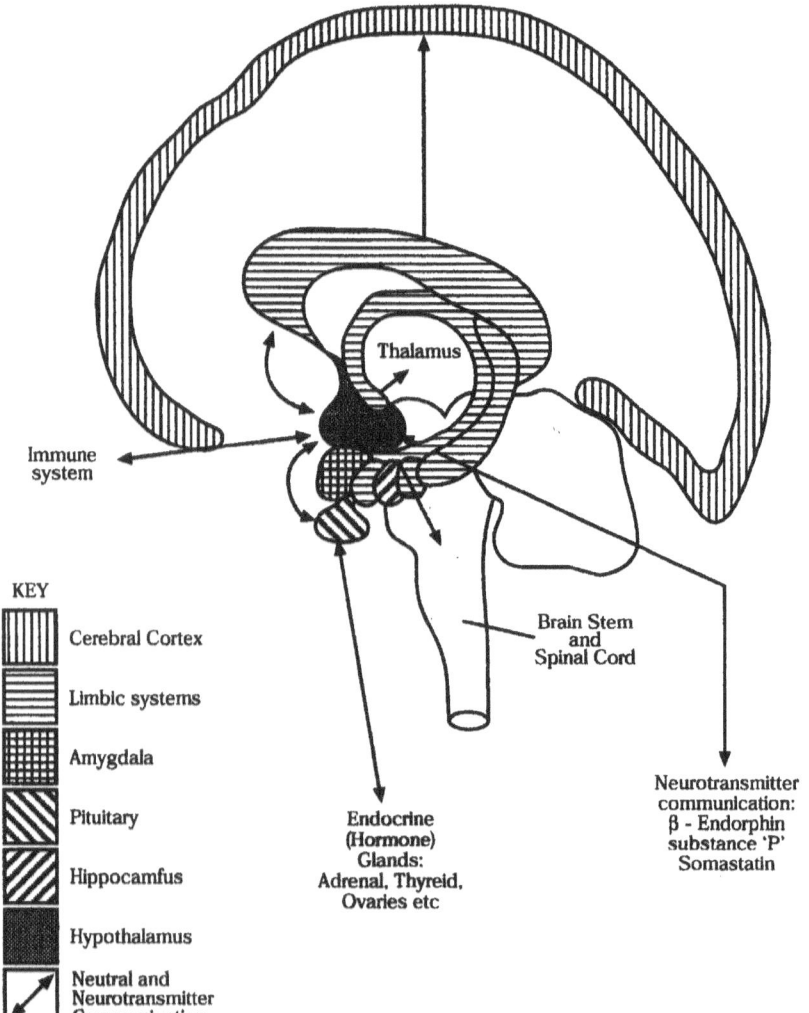

The hypothalamus can be compared to the central processing unit in a computer. This is the part of the brain which receives information from all other parts of the body and brain - from our senses of sight, hearing, touch, taste, and smell; from our pain sensors, from the balance centres of the brain, etc. This information is integrated with the corticolimbic part of the brain which includes memory and the information is reacted to, the highest priority being survival.

The hypothalamus has innumerable neural or nerve connections to other parts of the brain, amygdala, hippocampus, other brain structures and spinal cord to include the voluntary, as well as the involuntary, nervous systems, known respectively as the central nervous system (CNS) and the autonomic nervous system (ANS). However, that is not all. The hypothalamus also has influence over the pituitary gland via a hormonal system. The pituitary gland produces other hormones which signal the various target organs to produce their own specific hormones, such as thyroid hormone, oestrogen, cortisone, etc. There is yet another and very important message system, called 'neurotransmitters'. These are tiny protein particles or peptides that also have a specific message to give to various target organs, even single cells, which include the immune system, the white cells, T-killer cells, antibodies. The last time I read about them, about fifty neurotransmitters had been identified - but of course there are probably thousands, if not more. We are learning, every day.

So the hypothalamus acts as the real 'nerve centre' of the brain and according to the circumstances of any moment, issues forth a myriad of signals to all parts of the body, all in the interest of survival. We can compare this process to the battle management station on a naval missile cruiser. The commander sits before a great many screens which are monitored by his expert officers and other ranks. They will provide him with an up to date report of a given situation - surface radar to identify what ships are about and where; how many unidentified aircraft are about with their positions, speeds and headings. With all this information, the commander must make decisions under advisement and call the shots. He will decide on what action, if any, to take. He will issue commands to his gunnery officers, his weapons officers, his engine room and bridge. And he will be getting continuous feedback. Information is going backwards and forwards. In a battle situation, it is no easy task. But he must maintain the safety of his ship and crew as an effective fighting unit. The mind-body, today referred to as 'bodymind', connection is similar.

Information about pain or infection and so on causes a reaction. A thought or an emotion is also acted upon and so yet another 'mouthful' of a word is coined: psychoneuroimmunology, the integrated response of thought/emotion/nervous systems/immune system within the body. The full significance of this extended cascade is only now beginning to be appreciated. And the significance of a **thought** or an **emotion** in the development of disease is becoming more and more evident. We are aware today that many catastrophic diseases are preceded by a significant negative emotional event within two years of the onset of symptoms.

There are then two ways in which we can influence emotional disease and its consequences. We can identify the neurotransmitters involved and find a way to block them out - or indeed to enhance them. This is the goal of modern medicine and pharmacology. Or we can find the responsible thought or emotion and stop the rot at its source - this is the goal of hypnoanalysis.

One hopes that in time all the biochemical or neurotransmitter secrets will be discovered and put to effective use in the future. However, it is disheartening that the perceptions of this purely Newtonian approach ignore important factors. Every disease will have some final common pathway in terms of an alteration of the normal chemistry of body function - which technically may be called pathophysiology. But it is appropriate to consider the following:

Firstly, neurotransmitter dysfunction may in many cases be the result of a **thought** or an **emotion**, or a firmly imprinted belief, rather than the empirical result of a genetic code. More evidence is accumulating to confirm that it is these triggers which result in the opening of the genetic code gate. When this book was first published in the late 1990's it was believed that gene expression is controlled by the presence of specific activator 'pegs'. When the gene is turned on, RNA blueprint copies are made. Consider that it may well be a subconscious thought which triggers the peg for either a positive or a negative cascade in the cortico-limbic-hypothalamic-pituitary-end organ, immune and autonomic systems.

More recently advances in optogenetics suggest that neuroscientists may be able to influence memories to the extent of erasing 'bad' memories. Optogentics is a technique utilising light to control neurons and other cells which have been genetically modified by actuators to express light-sensitive ion channels. Currently the interest is in the possibility of treating Post Traumatic Stress Disorder (PTSD) - amazing science fiction becoming reality! Perhaps these techniques will prove the next greatest advance in neuropsychology yet there are ethical reservations. If we can erase or modify memories it raises the scary picture of mind-control for nefarious purposes. However, we already have an excellent method of treatment of PTSD in Medical Hypnoanalysis which continues to be largely ignored.

Nevertheless today there is an explosion of knowledge in the field of ***epigenetics*** which confirms previous speculation. Scientific journals are awash with the discoveries of these pioneers as they integrate the psyche, mind and body. Imagine the advantages of bringing this under the control of one's own will!

As an example, one line of thought is that insulin-dependent diabetes is believed to have a genetic basis and is precipitated by a viral infection which affects the insulin-producing pancreatic cells, or an immune antibody response to the insulin producing cells. As the production of insulin decreases, the body is unable to respond to a carbohydrate load and diabetes results with high levels of sugar. This is the scientific approach and the treatment would be to provide the patient with insulin by injection. While using medical hypnoanalysis to treat a diabetic patient's anxiety, Dr Thomas Ritzman described a case in which, as the anxiety was progressively resolved, the patient began to have low blood sugar episodes. Her insulin requirements were reducing - her normal dose of injected insulin was now too much, and her dose was reduced as treatment continued. By the time her anxiety had been cured, she was using no insulin at all - her diabetes had been cured too!

Was it Fear which acted as the trigger to precipitate her genetic code and disease? It certainly seems so.

Another diabetic patient I know developed the disease at the age of ten, within a year of a violent home invasion by armed burglars, during which time she and her family were terrorised. I am not suggesting that every diabetic can be cured with hypnosis, but it is clear that this warrants investigation - and perhaps there are other diabetics who could benefit.

A cautionary word - while it appears that some people's genetically predisposed disease can be altered, this does not mean that all genetic disorders can be treated. This notion is patently ridiculous. There is no possible way that Down's syndrome, or genetic damage due to exposure to toxins in the womb (eg fetal-alcohol syndrome) can be reversed. The latter term describes babies who are handicapped in varying degrees as the result of excessive alcohol use by the pregnant mother.

A further precautionary note - each patient should have a proper and appropriate medical examination to exclude organic disease, which may have a subconscious origin, but still requires treatment!

We need to remain objective and realistic about the patient as a whole.

CHAPTER FOUR

Psychosomatic Disease

The desire to take medicine is perhaps the greatest feature which distinguishes man from animals.
Sir William Osler;
Science and Immortality

If you believe Life to be fun, it very often is;
If you believe Life to be tough, it nearly always is.

As will be seen in case discussions, one has to try to determine whether an illness or disease is psychosomatic or not. Psychosomatic illness is described by Luban-Plozza and Poldinger as "disturbing physical symptoms that cannot be linked to any primary anatomic-pathological findings or pathological process, but which are a consequence, accompanying symptom of, or aspect of psychic, particularly emotional, processes." Coville, Costello and Rouke describe it as follows: "A psychosomatic disorder is the result of chronic or severe disruption of the delicate homeostatic balance of the body resulting from psychological stress." Generally, problems such as spastic colon and tension headaches are included in the psychosomatic spectrum. However, many of my patients with far more severe pathological processes like asthma and Lupus Erythematosus have been able to identify a definite subconscious cause ... and their disease has disappeared!

Now, what constitutes a psychosomatic illness? What potential is there to remove disease, and to greatly reduce the cost of treating a patient? The long-term medical costs of treating a Lupus patient, for example, may run into hundreds of thousands, if not millions, of Rands, especially if severe organ involvement such as kidney failure occurs. It would seem penny wise, pound foolish to ignore the potential of medical hypnoanalysis to cure such patients. Are Lupus and other similar diseases 'malignant' psychosomatic illnesses?

If a single patient has benefited from hypnoanalysis, may there not be similar relief for others? If this book excites only one or two academics and stimulates research, it will have been worth all the criticism I have received, all the rejections of important articles. An argument often put forth regarding Lupus and other connective tissue disorders is that we know that these illnesses can and do have spontaneous remissions and that their resolution by medical hypnoanalysis or some other modality is just such a remission. A renowned UK rheumatologist rejected one of my articles for this reason. The article was subsequently published by another journal.

My counter-argument is: if this is so, we need to examine what mind-body processes allowed the remission to occur. Was it not due to positive changes in the patients' spiritual or emotional behaviour and beliefs, with the principles of psychoneuro-immunology being applied subconsciously? If this is the case, there must be a strong argument to investigate a negative thought as being the cause of the disease in the first place, and manage it!

Furthermore, whatever future medicines or chemicals are developed and used to inhibit or stimulate the cascade described above, it is important to question whether the torpedo which causes the disease has already been fired. When prescribing a tranquiliser we are merely suppressing an emotion: the original problem remains - and is not available to the conscious mind. So, when the patient discontinues the drug and is later confronted by another 'threat', the symptoms are likely to recur. As my American colleague, the late Dr Dan Zelling, has said: "Anxiety is not a benzodiazepine-deficient disease!"

Dr Michael Meaney, of McGill University in Canada and who may be considered as a 'father' of epigenetics, has done some very telling experimental research. He separated some new-born rats from their mothers for fifteen minutes a day, and a second group of genetically identical babies for six hours a day. He found that the neurotransmitter receptors **and** the gene for the receptors were altered! The adult rats from the first group had more receptors and were less likely to be flooded with hormones like adrenalin during stress. The second group, however, had fewer receptors and were more likely to overproduce stress hormones. He found that early life experiences were so influential in the rats that they literally determined which receptor genes were turned on - and thus how many different types of receptors the brain actually produced! Clearly, the importance of genetics is shown to be secondary to the importance of early life experiences in certain circumstances. I believe that if similar research were to include the prenatal period, results would be similar.

All too often we see patients survive one crisis only to succumb to another ... and yet another. It is an interesting exercise to take a really good history from a patient and note the correlation of disease to emotional crises, whether the latter are admitted or denied. I know of one patient who had the following cascade: a ruptured berry aneurysm of an artery in the brain, which was successfully clipped in surgery, saving her life. This was followed by a perforated appendicitis with peritonitis. Having recovered from this, she developed an acute leukaemia to which she succumbed. All these crises occurred within a couple of years! Having experience in medical hypnoanalysis, one has to ask the question, did she have a subconscious belief of death - was her body merely conforming to that faulty belief?

Another patient had also, in her adult life, undergone a gastrectomy for a gastric ulcer from which she had a major bleed; severe pneumonia, a heart attack and a stroke as she became older. Each of these illnesses was associated with a preceding crisis in her marriage or nuclear family, and was accompanied by feelings of guilt and rejection. Each illness resulted, of course, in increased attention and caring.

I had a patient in general practice who developed pneumonia three years in succession: each year the timing of her illness coincided with the week her husband had died.

In the February 1997 issue of *Therapeutics* the problem of galactorrhoea is discussed. Galactorrhoea is the persistent discharge of milk or a milk-like secretion from the breast which is unrelated to pregnancy or feeding. In this article, emotional causes are entirely ignored. Pituitary tumours and prolactin are, however, examined in depth. Prolactin is the hormone produced by the pituitary gland which stimulates milk production in the breasts. I saw a patient in practice whose prolactin was ten times the normal maximum level, purely as a result of anxiety and I believe she and others like her are at risk of developing adenomas, tumours which may produce excessive prolactin.

My belief is that a great deal of medical practice is therefore crisis management. We appear to have lost our way in terms of truly preventive medicine. Is there an alternative? I believe there is. It is clear that we cannot divorce medicine from emotion, nor from spirituality. Ultimately, a holistic approach should be followed.

I read an article on irritable bowel syndrome (IBS) - spastic colon is part of this problem - in which the author questions whether it is indeed a psychosomatic problem or not. He cites studies that indicate that people with IBS have **less** anxiety than the general population. Herein lies the very crux of the problem of uninformed and blinkered medical thinking! Consider - the subconscious mind has chosen IBS as the proof of life, to deflect and minimise the anxiety. If it does this successfully and provides an adequate symptom, we should **expect** and can predict that there will be less anxiety! The subconscious mind has achieved its goal!

When the mind has concluded that there is no longer any conscious or subconscious meaning to life, when all purpose and hope are lost, and survival is no longer an issue, the physical body will conform to that belief in whichever way is appropriate or convenient. These were the words of the thinkers in medical hypnoanalysis, Drs William Bryan and Thomas Ritzman.

To a doctor using all his resources to save his patient, it is akin to plugging a leak in the dyke with a finger, whilst knowing full well that there are a dozen other potential leaks nearby - but just out of reach. It is frustrating and often exasperating. Today, in many cases, these potential leaks are not out of reach.

One of the methods that may be used is the modality of Medical Hypnoanalysis which preceded work in 'primal therapy' by Janov, as well as work by Grof` and others. I believe it is a far more logical, systematic and thorough approach, than these. It is not based on a new psychological theory, but rather makes use of existing psychological therapeutic techniques. Medical hypnoanalysis needs to be distinguished from traditional hypnoanalysis, which is not nearly as directed: while utilising regression as the major tool it does not have the advantage of the concepts of the diagnoses of medical hypnoanalysis. Traditional hypnoanalysis follows the therapeutic processes of for example, the psychobiological therapy of Meyer or the principles of Rogerian psychotherapy, directive therapy etc. Medical hypnoanalysis may indeed utilise these psychotherapy principles but in a more effective manner. Importantly, it recognises the essential spiritual nature of humankind.

In brief, it is a structured, short term method of identifying the original threatening events that were associated with powerful negative emotional imprints - the original thoughts and emotions which form the basis of learned subconscious responses to future events in life. The process is undertaken in hypnotic trance and is aimed at conscious realisation of these events and feelings, removing the inappropriate negative beliefs that resulted, and replacing them with positive beliefs, rehabilitating the patient towards a new and healthier response to stressors.

One should recognise that our society bombards us continuously with certain messages which can be, and are, assimilated into our basic response patterns. The film and TV industry is an example of such exposure, as are the words we hear from our parents, relatives, teachers and ministers of religion, from sports heroes. We hear negative phrases such as "he gives me a pain in the arse", "you are a headache to me", "heartache", "you don't have a leg to stand on" and many others. Subliminally we learn at least two things from these. Firstly, that we are responsible for other people's deepest responses. Secondly, we learn to respond in the same way, subconsciously. A colleague of mine in the USA developed a cancer of his thigh with the underlying subconscious belief that he did not 'have a leg to stand on'! Another developed cancer of the bladder with the thought "that pisses me off". There are numerous other examples, and if we want to be a little facetious, maybe we develop our painful strangulated piles because we have, or we allow others to give us, a pain right there!

In the Newtonian objective world, each of us lives out our lives in what we perceive to be the concrete reality. The fact is that our reactions are based on firmly imprinted beliefs established very early in life. They may and often do begin, during intrauterine life, during the birth experience and the immediate postnatal period. For example, a person who is hyperventilating in a panic attack is simply going through the actions of the 'being-born' child with a compulsion to breathe in the presence of a dire asphyxiating threat to his survival. It is nothing more than that.

As Fritjof Capra, Ritzman and many others have said, the problem that modern medicine faces is that it is still back in the Newtonian-Cartesian world view - a philosophy from which the science of physics escaped with Einstein's Theory of Relativity, Planck's Theory of Quantum Mechanics and Heisenberg's Uncertainty Principle, even though these are 'stumbling' after Chiao's work on the speed of light. Much coverage is currently being given to this in the medical press, by authors here and internationally, too numerous to mention by name. My perception of this body of work is that it ignores the obvious - the subconscious and the spiritual self. These words sound very erudite, but do not contribute a great deal to the underlying understanding and the practicalities of treating a patient. While the fiddler plays, Rome - the patient - burns ... but there are already many answers. Some action is being taken by certain doctors and psychologists who are prepared to work at the coalface in new territory, and who have that extraordinary curiosity and faith.

A pregnant mother may be anxious for any number of reasons or be feeling guilt or shame. She may not have wanted to be pregnant at that time due to problems with her partner, or because of financial difficulties. She may be ill. She may be aware that because of her own emotional turmoil, she is just not ready for a pregnancy. Whatever the cause, today we know that from early on in the pregnancy the foetus is aware of maternal feelings and may be influenced by her responses and by other outside events.

This does not imply 'fault or blame' on the part of the mother, or the father. It acknowledges that we are all vulnerable humans and react to the perceptions of our own earliest experiences. It suggests that forgiveness should ultimately be relatively easy - once understanding has been allowed ... and forgiveness is important to healing in many people.

However, in the absence of consistent maternal love the foetus may become confused as to its purpose and meaning. Often the foetus feels responsibility for the mother's predicament, initiating guilt. Remember that the foetus has no sense of logic, or a database to which it can refer. It must react to what it is experiencing - and the only logic that subconscious has is related to survival. It thinks like this: does this event support my life, or does it lead to death. There is a sense of profound loneliness ... of rejection. It begins to question its right to simply be. Anxiety as to future survival - both physical and spiritual - ensues. All meaning and purpose may be lost as is its vital connection with mother, the family, and the universe at large - its sense of love and self, of soul and God. The subconscious is compelled to do something to ensure survival - and often there is a 'switching off', a dissociation from the pain, and a retreat to a limbo wherein the pain is no longer felt ... a dying. This is not a metaphorical dying - it is emotional and spiritual death, and presents as depression and other problems later.

With this devastation and uncertainty, the baby is then confronted with the birth experience, which is almost universal in its terror. This is the perception of the child: the opinion of the doctor or mother matters little and is irrelevant. The 'easiest' of deliveries can be experienced by the baby as a catastrophic threat to physical survival. Low oxygen levels during contractions or when the cord is trapped between the baby and the birth canal wall, result in a chemically induced apprehension. There is a feeling of suffocation, extreme pressure on the head and chest accompanied by pain ... and a fear of impending death. The flight or fight survival response is initiated by the subconscious with the release of adrenalin. This great struggle leaves the baby exhausted and nauseous. Any further delay results in hopelessness and surrender to the supposed inevitability of death.

Delivery by elective Caesarian section may also be traumatic. The baby is precipitated into a colder and more threatening environment from the known warm, safe womb. The effects of the anaesthetic given to the mother are not just chemical; the baby is aware that mother is suddenly 'not there'. A later chapter on Post Traumatic Stress Disorder details the experience of our patient who was delivered by an elective Caesarian section - that is, a planned, non-emergency operation.

With the physical survival of this terrifying experience, the alleviating life-assuring factor is maternal bonding - **love**. Should this be of a poor quality, delayed or absent, the child's doubts are confirmed. Removal from mother to an incubator or simply to a cradle intensifies the loneliness, aggravating the separation experience. Should the baby have mucus in its throat requiring suctioning, this intensifies and aggravates the fear - it causes a choking sensation. A delay in feeding is similarly threatening. All these brief descriptions are typical, every-day findings in a medical hypnoanalyst's office.

Dr Don Ebrahim came to the same conclusions in England, in his work with clinical hypnosis - and he terms it 'Traumatic Separation Theory'. He is absolutely correct in saying that any **future** separation may well be deemed by the subconscious to be equally if not more threatening to survival.

Dr Herbert Strean, who co-authored the book *The Severed Soul* with Lucy Freeman, states that "I have never witnessed a case [of schizophrenia] where there was a consistently loving environment in childhood." However, we need to again extend our field of vision to our knowledge of the prenatal period.

It is already becoming clear that the baby may be confronted with different threats in terms of survival. There is a distinction between physical and spiritual survival. Patients who have difficulty in accepting their inherent spiritual energy and rightful place in the universe are the ones whose prognosis is the poorest.

The spiritual self is beyond the probing fingers of Newtonian objectivity or Einsteinian subjectivity - indeed it is beyond quantum uncertainty. It cannot be measured, except perhaps intangibly by the degree of love one is able to generate and give. Science, in this aspect, is rigidly limited. How do we reconcile science with spirituality?

Consider that time, space, all matter and all energy were created in a single cataclysmic release of energy some fourteen billion years ago. Astrophysicists cannot agree even on this figure. Be that as it may, this is the Big Bang Theory, or Biblical Genesis – whichever one wishes to accept or reject. Both are the same. Prior to that there was ... nothing - nothing measurable. Everything we can measure with instruments today resulted from this release of energy, every sub-nuclear particle, all forces, every star ... every rock ... every living entity. We are all part of this vast energy force. We interact with it, knowingly or not. A dynamic continuous interchange exists within this pool, at cosmic and individual levels. One's own body is in a state of dynamic exchange, atom for atom. The atoms one is born with are no longer part of one's body. One has shed cells and atoms, absorbed and integrated new ones. Physiologically the body is renewed on average every seven years, more slowly with the ageing process. Yet there is a constant - one's spirit. Every culture throughout history has as its basis this perception of spirituality, of the connection to the universal energy. This is not New Age Thinking!

In Genesis, God says: "Let there be light"… and there was light. Astrophysicists have mathematically demonstrated that the first three minutes of the known universe consisted of light – photon energy. Thomas Ritzman wrote a wonderful article based on his experiences and Dr William Bryan's work, in which he explains that this energy from which everything came, is the first tangible expression of God. As nothing we know is created without a preceding thought, it follows that behind this Divine energy, there is thought, Divine thought. And since the ever-evolving universe has progressed into a more and more organised system, resulting in at least the semi-intelligent human race, there must be a purpose to all this. We do not have to know what that purpose is to feel comfortable as an integral **part** of that plan. We **are** by the very fact of our being. These three expressions of God manifest in us through the energy of **love**. Love is that energy most required in all of us.

One may speculate on what one discovers in examining and stripping the human body down to its constituent atoms and beyond. An atom is a system of balanced electrical charges and forces - primordial energy - a system collectively arranged in such a way that produces and is produced by ... thought? To be grand, Divine thought ... a spiritual belonging - that stirring deep inside when one looks up at a sky full of stars on a moonless desert night; the yearning for an unknown common home and a strong, undeniable identification with and love for a universal spirituality. Rejection of this in the objective Newtonian macrocosm must result in a breakdown of order in the instruments of that energy ... mind and body.

In the pure physical sense, a completely isolated system has a tendency to pass from order to disorder - described in physics as the 'entropy' of the system. The larger the system's entropy, the greater its state of disorder. In its physical interaction with its environment, such a system causes the release of heat ... and heat increases entropy.

When a memory is consolidated, and a thought conceived, a tiny amount of energy in the form of heat is released in the activation of a neurone by neurotransmitters. As heat increases, entropy increases. The conflicting perceptions of reality and imprinted memories result in the release of more energy with the increased activity of the brain ... disorder increases. All living organisms, by temporarily maintaining their own order, increase their environmental system's entropy. Ultimately an homogenous inactive state must result: an all-encompassing black hole perhaps, or an existential vacuum.

This poses the question that if the universal entropy is arrowed towards ultimate chaos and maximum disorder, as the physicists tell us is so, are we ourselves on a path of inevitable and ultimate disorder? A frightening thought - but it is frightening only when one is bound and limited by the objectivity of Newtonian science, by the uncertainty of Heisenberg's principle, and of what occurs in a black hole, where even quantum mechanics becomes nonsensical; when physicists, in mathematical models, get to within one second to the minus thirtieth power after the Big Bang. Most pertinently, in humankind, it is frightening only because of the uncertainty of what happens to us after we die.

Present knowledge limits our perception of the universe to that of an isolated physical system. However, Stephen Hawking, acknowledged as one of the finest scientific minds since Einstein, wondered whether, in terms of the theory of quantum mechanics, the energy trapped in a black hole 'goes off into another universe'. Accident or Design? Hawking has also stated that the universe is so fine-tuned as to seem to have purpose.

He has stated that had the charge on the electron been the tiniest bit greater or less that no life could ever have evolved because no star could ever have formed. Even a supernova - a catastrophic event indeed - has purpose. It adds heavier atoms to the resources of a galaxy, without which there could be no organic life. We would not have been here to read, write, laugh, cry or love.

Our narrow perspectives are what threaten us, our own reactions to events which allow us to fear the future. Why do we worry? Anxiety springs from the same fear that began in the birth experience, compounding the doubts of our spiritual reality first perceived in the uterus. All fear is the fear of death, be it physical or spiritual death. It hampers us and prevents us from truly living our lives.

If we aspire to the best ideal in medicine - truly preventive medicine - then we must consider the emotions, thoughts and ideas that result in many diseases. We must consider the spirit.

To conserve energy, to reduce the rate of our individual progressive disorder, should we not be paying more attention to the original negative thoughts and imprints? Promoting order at this point would encourage healing at all levels. To do this is beyond Newtonian and Einsteinian physics, it is beyond our concepts of quantum mechanics - it is in the realm of our spirituality: a fact known to, and used by, our distant ancestors.

Man's inherent desire for truth is the source of all learning and scientific endeavour, and the quality which sets man apart from the animals is an aspiration towards spirituality. The driving force is love, a seeking for fusion with the source of our existence, and thereby ultimate meaning.

Astrophysicists have long sought a grand unified field theory, which would unite Newtonian, Einsteinian and quantum theory. Applying this to the human sciences, we require an improved diagram, or map. We can now look at a third diagram for a more complete picture of the dynamics between mind and body - and perhaps provide a deeper perspective of the disease process. This will also enable those in the healing professions to see the patient in a fuller dimension, as William Osler prescribed.

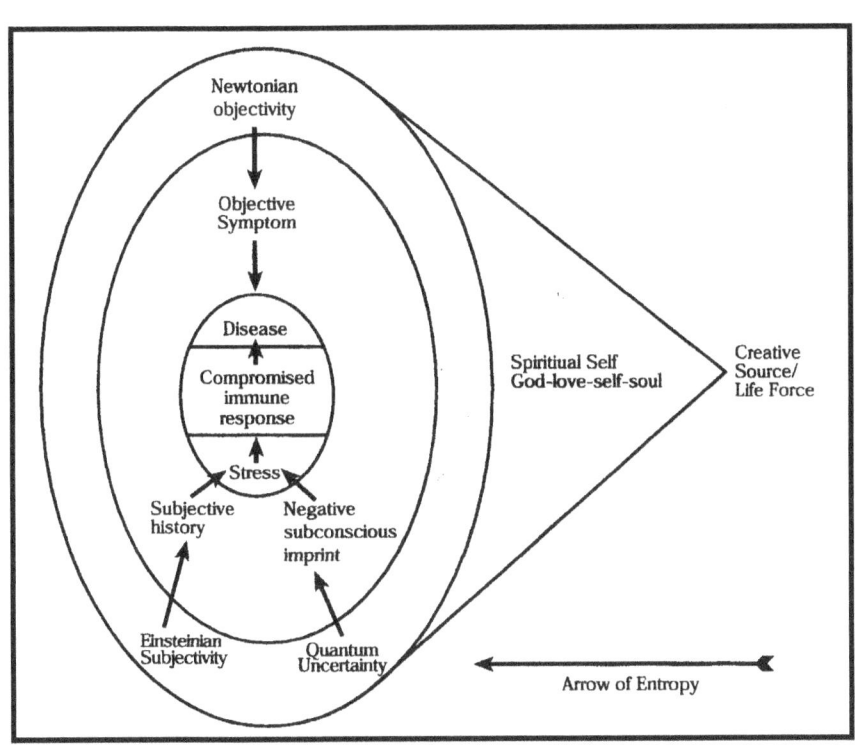

Behind the psychodynamics and behind the physical manifestations of disease, lies the spectrum of one's spirituality - a key to many problems we encounter. It is now easier to ask the question "why is this patient having this problem?"

Professor Sam Fehrsen, former editor of the journal *South African Family Practice* correctly pointed out to me that some readers may feel uncomfortable with this concept; that, as a creation of God we are indeed a part of God, a part of the all-pervading infinite multi-universal energy. The Collective Consciousness of Jung. Robert Heinlein, in his novel *Stranger in a Strange Land* has his human character born and brought up on Mars, to later greet Earthlings with the exclamation "Thou art God". Small wonder that it was banned in the then atavistic and rigidly Calvinist South Africa! It may be construed as blasphemous, and this point is of great importance, because it has to do with the most destructive of all the emotions - guilt. Later, we will spend some time examining guilt, its causes and effects on the human condition.

Meanwhile however, the ability to say '**I love me**' is synonymous with saying 'I belong here. I have a purpose and meaning.' Eric Berne calls it 'I'm OK'. Viktor Frankl - another remarkable man, wrote: 'Despair equals suffering without meaning. D=S-M.' He created an entire psychotherapy – logotherapy - with one basic premise: **meaning**. I put the following question to doubters: If one cannot love oneself, wholly and unconditionally, how is it possible to truly love God or anyone, for that matter? As the creation of God, it follows that to love Him, we **must** love ourselves. This was the fundamental message of Christ and the Old Testament: "Love others as you love yourself".

Any other "love" is merely a quest for a return of respect and attention, a quest to find love from someone **else** that will confirm to us 'Yes, I am safe. I am loveable. I am a worthy person.' This is not love. It is a parody of love. The only 'soul mate' that there is, is yourself ... as part of the infinite energy, as part of God. Those unfortunate people who are eternally seeking **the** marriage partner are doomed for this very reason. Instead of looking to the outside for fulfilment, they should be looking within. Add to this group those even more unfortunate people who become terrified of 'God' as a result of what they perceived or were taught as children, one has an idea of the huge proportion of the population who are in trouble.

Consider those well publicised ladies and gentlemen of fame and fortune, who are into their seventh or eighth marriage. Sure, it's immature behaviour. It's 'immature' because somewhere they probably got stuck in childhood looking for love from an unattainable source. They're still looking for love outside of themselves. And no amount of talking will help - it is an unfulfilled **subconscious** need. They need to be taken back to the source and to understand that the love has always been there, inside themselves.

In my earlier, more ignorant days, I would receive letters from various psychologists to whom I had referred a patient. Letters which said: 'when she finds someone to love her, she'll be OK.' Oh dear. That may well be ... **but**, what happens to her if 'he' runs off with another woman, or dies? Her source and purpose of life has gone, she crashes right back into her own oblivion. She is more vulnerable than before! 'He and she' are of course interchangeable. 'I love me' is the very essence of living - three of the six most important words in the universe. Unfortunately, much of our growing years seem to deflect us from this truth. This book is about those mechanisms, those perceptions. The new map puts our quest into perspective. So, to return to our basic scientific format: If we are not following this map, we need to ask

- How can I begin?
- What can help me escape the trap?
- Why is it not happening?
- Where do I begin?
- When can I start?

The ethos of the World Health Organisation is 'to enable people to increase their control over and improve their health'. If one accepts that many problems are based on learned subconscious survival responses, our calling is surely to help people understand these, why they arose and then facilitate **change.** The answers lie in each of us. All that is required is the decision, and that should not be difficult - we have choices today that we did not have as a foetus or as an infant. The essential element is a genuine desire to change.

It is up to ... you.

CHAPTER FIVE

Medical Hypnoanalysis

To fear love is to fear life, and those who fear life are already three parts dead.
Bertrand Russel; Marriage and Morals, 1929.

We can now examine medical hypnoanalysis, which is the modality I consider to be the most effective. It is effective because it is logical: it makes sense not just to me, but to the **patient**, who after all is the important figure. Furthermore it is also the only modality which includes the inherent spirituality of man as a fundamental issue.

This is certainly not meant to be a text book - indeed, I have deliberately excluded the technical issues, lest they be misused. Nevertheless, it is necessary to gain some insight into the philosophies underlying medical hypnoanalysis in order to begin to understand oneself, and this book. It is an interesting journey.

One of the most basic aspects of medical hypnoanalysis is that it does not prejudge any person or any event. It does not presuppose some failure or inadequacy in a patient. Rather it suggests that some illness is determined by the person's learned **survival** response to his perceptions of an event, or events.

To understand this, one needs to realise that subconsciously we live and survive according to a scale of priorities, which is called the Order of Importance. The 'least' important level of survival is that of sexual drive. Without sex, there would be no intercourse, no babies and the human race would disappear from the earth in one generation. This instinct ensures the survival of the human race. Next on the scale is territory - the space and field of operation required for survival, just as a pride of lions has a defined territory in which to hunt and reproduce. One up from this is physical survival - food, water and, oxygen. We are now getting to more critical survival issues. The following level is that of mind survival - one's esteem or respect of self, and esteem of others, one's ability to think and create. Ultimately, there is spiritual survival - one's sense of the connection of Self in terms of love, soul and God - continuation of the spirit. So:

7. Sex	.....	Species survival
6. Territory	.....	Socio-economic survival
5. Food }		
4. Water }	.....	Physical survival
3. Oxygen }		
2. Self esteem/ethics	.....	Mind or Ego survival
1. Self/*Love*/soul/God	.....	Spiritual survival

Thus, when someone presents to me with say, a personality disorder, in which it is clear from the history that he is functioning extremely well sexually, making a mint of money at the socio-economic level and pumping iron at the gym, I know his **real** problem lies at a higher level: this is where I will look for clues, because his survival problem is either at the mind or spiritual levels. He has 'died' or accepted death subconsciously at one of these levels and hence can only function consistently at a lesser level.

Most importantly, this survival response has its **origin** in a very powerful **emotional** event, usually early in life. An equally important issue is that of ... **perceptions**. For example, a mother might say "that was the easiest baby I ever delivered" and her doctor will confirm that. "Oh yes. Very straightforward - the baby's APGAR was 9 in just one minute." That may be true for them - but it is not relevant to the baby! Because what the **baby** perceives of this birth process is usually something entirely different.

A colleague of mine referred his son to me and advised me that his birth was quick and easy - just half an hour. In regression, we spent two hours helping him through! This is unusual in therapy - most often the regression is over within five or ten minutes. However, at the time of birth, it may seem an endless struggle to the baby. How often has one sat in a lesson or a lecture for only sixty minutes but which **seemed** to last hours and hours? If one can feel like this in a non-threatening environment, how has one reacted under real stress?

Memory is not perfect. Indeed, we have already seen in our explanation of hypnosis that a person can lie and confabulate in trance. Further, what the patient perceives may have no bearing on the reality of the event at all. For example, I had a patient with a phobia for water; she also had problems in dealing with relationships. In hypnoanalysis, it became apparent that her problems originated from when she was just six weeks old. Her mother was bathing her in the baby bath and she was slippery with soap. She slipped out of her mother's arms into the water, face down. She had two immediate perceptions. One, "I am going to die because I can't breathe" and two, "mother did it to me". She was both terrified and angry ... her trust in those around her began to falter. The **facts** were of course, that her mum did not deliberately drop her - there was no malice. Also, mum immediately picked her up, hugged her and soothed her. However, to the patient things were very different ... and she never forgave her mother. Not until she was able to go back and see the event in a different light.

So it is important to realise that we are dealing with the perceptions of events. From a therapeutic point of view, these **perceptions** cause many faulty beliefs - they are what need to be examined. The facts are of secondary importance. I am neither judge nor jury in terms of commenting on the validity of what really happened. Mostly, what the patient remembers is very accurate - and this has been verified time and time again - but not always. Hence the title of this book – "Prisoners of our Perceptions"!

Another advantage of the modality of medical hypnoanalysis is that it is short term treatment - most patients can be successfully treated in twenty or so sessions. Traditionally, 'analysis' has been synonymous with a very lengthy process - years. In comparison to psychoanalysis, it is decidedly more rapid - ten to twenty times more so. This is of course time- and cost-saving. The reason for this is the nature of the phenomenon of hypnosis - we can communicate with both the conscious and the subconscious mind and it is in the subconscious that the answers are to be found. The subconscious mind **knows** what the score is. A patient often says to me at the first interview: "I know it is silly and even stupid to feel this way, but **I can't seem to help myself**! How true - and I tell them that if they **did** know the reason they would not have come to me in the first place - they would have solved the problem themselves!

Why should that be? Let's explore ...

The conscious mind is responsible for our ability to think logically - to reason, to understand ... and to make the decisions. The subconscious mind is responsible for memory, for emotions, for monitoring our body functions, and for controlling the latter; it is responsible for our survival instincts, our creativity, etc. The subconscious is extremely limited in logic. It has been termed the 'all-powerful idiot', while the conscious mind has been called the 'impotent genius'. The only logic that the subconscious has is at the level of survival - it sees each and every event in one of two ways ... does this support my life? Or, does it lead to my death? Furthermore, it is compelled to **act** on this - **survival** is the key. Survival is everything.

Let us examine memory. From the time the brain is able to receive any messages through the senses, it records our history. These memories remain there until we die ... they can only be removed if that part of the brain is destroyed by trauma, disease or surgery ... which **is** trauma. Most memories are positive and good or at least neutral - no big deal. However, some memories are negative, fewer still are **very** negative. Based on this record of our experience, we develop a learned, automatic - subconscious - habitual pattern of responding to the world. We respond in the way we think (cognitively), the way we feel (emotionally), and in the way we act (behaviourally).

So far so good. However, there is a problem. The subconscious has the ability to **block off** any memory ... to hide it from the conscious mind. This is always in the interests of survival ... to prevent a particular perceived threat to survival from causing distress to the individual.

One of these hidden traumatic memories is the key to the patient's problem - the **'real problem'**. This blocking off usually occurs when the patient is still very young, before a reasonable level of maturity, logic and independence has been attained. For example, it is as if the subconscious says: "you are now so filled with fear, or guilt, that you cannot function. I will block off this memory so that you can still go on ... even though less effectively at some levels. It is better than experiencing these feelings. I'll give you a lesser symptom instead." These unavailable memories may be due to a later experience in life - for example in response to a rape, or major trauma - but usually they have their origin early in life. For example, I had one thirty-plus year old patient whose real problem occurred at the age of seventeen: she had no conscious recollection of the traumatic rape she was subjected to at all!

If I were to ask you, the reader, to describe your second birthday party, you probably would be unable to tell me a thing. However, if you were in hypnosis, and your subconscious agreed to go back to that day, you would recall in detail everything ... or most things. The type of cake and how it tasted ... what you were wearing ... who was there ... whether you blew the candles out or not ... and even better, what presents you received.

So, we do **not** have automatic access to **all** of our memories ... and there lies the problem. Which is just as well, for if we were continually bombarded with everything from our life we would be psychotic: this is protective of our normal functioning. It is only the **conscious** mind that can use reason, logic and understanding and make the decision to **change** the old automatic responses, **but** it doesn't know what the problem is - the real problem is buried in the subconscious mind! The subconscious mind knows **exactly** what the problem is, but cannot do anything about it. It is still locked into an historical and out-dated survival mode ... it doesn't know the danger is over and done with, unnecessary. It **must**, it is compelled to, continue a survival effort.

Worse still, any later event which powerfully re-enacts the **same** feelings of anxiety, fear or guilt ... will result in an **intensification** of the survival response. Such an event is again seen by the subconscious as life-threatening ... it **must** provide a wall of protection, and it is this wall of protection which is the symptom the patient presents with. It is this automatic response of thinking, feeling and behaving which is the symptom – whether its migraine, spastic colon, anxiety or whatever.

Clearly, it is necessary to identify these events - particularly the 'real problem' and remove the negative emotional impact they had. If this can be done, it is a great deal easier to change the old negative responses to positive ones. Sometimes, the patient's subconscious does this automatically once the issue has been confronted ... but often, the patient needs to be helped with the process.

The way a symptom develops is not unlike the way in which a person develops an allergy. It is also a negative conditioning, resulting from past experience. For example, when I was five years old I was set upon by a Dalmatian dog. Later, as a general practitioner, I was requested to do a house call and despite the presence of the householder, his Rottweiler took a healthy piece from my lower calf. This negative conditioning resulted in my reticence to do another house call at that home, or any home with large dogs! This is 'conditioning'! Pavlov's dog was conditioned to salivate with the bell ringing to announce food was coming.

To provide an allergy analogy, let us consider a person who is allergic to penicillin for example. We can even accept that this person has an inherited susceptibility from his mother or father, or perhaps from the combination of their genetic contributions, which makes him potentially allergic to penicillin. The first time he is given penicillin, he usually has no reaction whatsoever. Why not? Well, he has had no previous exposure, he has not yet built up any antibodies to penicillin - so no reaction will occur. However, he has now become **sensitised**, which means that when he receives penicillin again, he does have some antibodies, and so he gets an allergic reaction, a symptom for the first time - he gets a rash, which is not too bad, nor does it last for long. This second exposure increases not only the speed with which his body will produce antibodies, but the amount it will produce. So, the third time he has penicillin, he gets a rash **and** perhaps starts wheezing with mild asthma. His antibody response is becoming more pronounced and the reaction time is shorter. The fourth time or the hundredth time - depending on how long it takes for him - he may have a catastrophic reaction with a rash, severe asthma, respiratory and cardiovascular collapse ... his blood pressure drops and without urgent medical attention, he may even die in anaphylactic shock.

In the same way we can use the analogy of 'emotional antibodies'. Please note there is no such thing as 'emotional antibodies' - this tautological example serves only to demonstrate how a symptom can develop. Again, it is accepted that the patient may have a genetic or inherited predisposition to anxiety, fear or guilt. The first time that he is exposed to an event which involves anxiety, fear or guilt, he has no symptom at all. This is called the **Initial Sensitising Event** or **ISE**. He has become **sensitised**. The degree of this sensitisation will depend on how intense that event was, and how intensely he reacted to it - we talk of the 'emotional voltage' of the event. The second time he experiences a similar event, his 'antibodies' now result in a symptom, which again is usually mild and temporary. Naturally enough, this event is called the **Symptom Producing Event** or **SPE**. With his increased responsiveness however, the third time he is exposed to a similar event, his symptoms get worse and last longer. This is known as the **Symptom Intensifying Event** or **SIE,** and he may experience several more over some years; each time his symptoms worsen - until the symptom may become 'permanent'.

Importantly, the ISE represents his **real problem** - and is **not** recalled by the conscious mind, until he is given the opportunity to go back to that time in hypnotic trance. When this is done, he can utilise his logical mind, maturity and experience to see that the problem is now a thing of the past - it should not affect him in the present. However, his subconscious mind **does not yet know** that the danger has passed - it cannot think logically. So the patient who fell into the bath at six weeks of age is likely to react with the same thoughts, feelings and actions in the future, and with each subsequent exposure to being in water or have water pouring on her from a shower her symptoms get worse. When she was able under hypnosis to go back in time and realise firstly that she survived that crisis and that today that baby bath is probably too small for both her feet, she is able to defuse the impact of the original event.

Consequently, her subconscious no longer needs to provide the adrenalin to ensure survival. Her anxiety about water disappears, especially if we are able to speed up the change from old automatic negative responses and replace them with an automatic **positive** response. This is most easily and effectively achieved by the use of direct suggestion in trance, or by the use of metaphors and so on.

The therapist must identify these significant events and remove their impact. Should this not be done, the result is often merely an exchange of one symptom for another. For example, let us imagine a person who stops smoking. The smoking habit was a symptom provided by the subconscious mind for a specific purpose and without this 'protection' there is still a need for a 'proof of life'. Instead of smoking, this person begins to gain weight - the subconscious is orally providing a protective layer of fat in lieu of the sucking in of air and oxygen that indicates 'I am still alive'.

How do we go about identifying these events? This is not too difficult in the majority of patients and we use a medical model - hence the term '**medical**' hypnoanalysis. When a patient visits a doctor with a sore throat, the first thing he will do is take a reasonable **history**. He will ask how long the throat has been sore, whether there has been coughing or a fever or not, and so on. Thus the first stage in medical hypnoanalysis is a history - a **very** detailed history, which may take up to an hour. We are searching for all the clues that the patient can give from his **conscious** mind - and very often he doesn't realise the significance of what he is saying, or of his body language, or even of the words he uses ... all of these may be significant and the medical hypnoanalyst is trained to focus on and note these things. They assist us in identifying the events and in making a presumptive *subconscious* diagnosis.

These are descriptive in nature and not only do they help **explain** the cause and nature of the symptom they are easily understood by the patient - enabling him to make real changes in his life.

There are only six such subconscious diagnoses, which together or singly put the symptom into an understandable perspective for the patient - who has to make the changes in his thinking. Formal psychiatric or medical diagnoses do not help much in this process. In fact, they sometimes give the patient a sense of hopelessness, of being 'labelled'. This is not my comment - it is a common response of patients who now 'see the light'. Indeed, the legal system recognises that a formal diagnosis may result in serious consequences for a patient. For example, the patient with migraine described earlier after his analysis **knew** that his headache actually was the result of a fear of death, and guilt. He was no longer afraid of dying a physical death in the birth canal, - he had really been afraid of **spiritual** death by having love and acceptance removed from him by his parents! He was afraid of God's judgement after he died – to heaven or hell? His subconscious could not differentiate between a spiritual or physical threat but was compelled to act. Previously, the diagnosis 'migraine' had consigned him to hopelessness. He is aware today that his 'migraine' was simply a symptom of an emotional and spiritual problem.

Let us briefly examine these diagnoses.

CHAPTER SIX

The Subconscious Diagnoses

1. The Prenatal Experience or PNE

    I'm a stranger and afraid, in a world I never made.
    AE Housman; Last Poems, 1922.

The prenatal experience, as its name clearly suggests, is the experience of the fetus while still in the womb. Most people, professionals and non-professionals, become critical when this subject is broached. Many become immediately aggressive and ridicule the notion that a baby in the womb has any awareness. They turn away in disgust ... and none will explain to me their reaction. Interesting.

We are aware today that from a scientific point of view the baby can be and is influenced by many stimuli. It has the ability to at least hear and touch, to sense differences in light and colour. The literature puts this ability from about twenty-eight weeks in the uterus. Our experience in hypnotic regression, confirmed by mothers in later interviews, is that these abilities can and do occur much earlier, especially in terms of **emotion**. There also appears to be an extrasensory perception in the relationship between mother and child which is largely the property of the baby.

One example is the patient who in a regression to fourteen weeks in the womb *(in utero)* became extremely agitated, fearful and pale while sitting on the chair in trance. In her regression, the womb around her was contracting, she was aware of her mother being in distress and she was extremely frightened of dying. Of course, she did not know what was happening. She then reported that she felt very dizzy and nauseous.

After this session, she contacted her mother who confirmed that at exactly that stage of pregnancy she had had a threatened miscarriage. Mother had been hospitalised and given an intravenous infusion of alcohol and ipratroprium which is a medication for asthma, but also helpful in reducing the irritability of the uterine muscle. What the patient experienced in the womb was drunkeness, a lowered blood pressure as well as a rising fear of impending disaster! Later in her life, when confronted with any threatening situation, she was apt to become very pale and anxious, dizzy and nauseous ... sometimes to the extent of vomiting. Clearly, she was responding from a subconscious level with the feelings she had experienced in the womb.

Another example, perhaps more significant in terms of the right to life, was the patient who was also very fearful of dying because her mother and father were considering an abortion. This ongoing discussion took place at just ten weeks of pregnancy! This patient insisted on an interview with her parents in my presence. The parents denied the allegation, not surprisingly, but after some lengthy, careful and painful discussion admitted to their original intent.

A fetus responds not only to its local environment, but also to the external environment. Babies are aware of parental arguments, sounds, music, grandparents and others. They are also aware of positive influences ... most especially in terms of **love** and acceptance.

A best-seller in America written by a minister of religion and his wife advocates the dictum "spare the rod and spoil the child". They go so far as to say that children are inherently naughty or bad, and that they require this sort of discipline. In our experience in medical hypnoanalysis, this is not only wrong, but dangerous - how many parents and would-be parents have been influenced by this? How many children will suffer the consequences? Ultimately, it is humanity which will endure generations of children who have a conduct disorder and who may become psychopaths.

To the fertilised egg, there are no problems. To the developing fetus, there are no problems. Indeed, I routinely regress patients to a time before maternal awareness of the pregnancy - and I find that the majority of patients are aware of light and a serenity beyond words ...

this is pure spiritual existence, a blissful state which is what the good Lord intended. I detect no evil at this time. That a minister of religion does not recognise this is quite an indictment. An indictment, I hasten to add, not of religion in general, but of our individual fallability. The perception of an individual's 'badness' or 'wrongness' is a faulty belief established by the baby's awareness of maternal or external factors.

I cannot criticise the notion - that children are basically bad - strongly enough, the emotion I feel is one of sadness. Babies are thinking, feeling beings long before they are born ... and may act out movements in their distress - they respond cognitively, emotionally and behaviourally, though their logic is limited. The sooner we recognise the fetus as a sentient being the better for Humankind.

A fetus exposed to a negative environment and then to the folly of what this best-seller recommends, is in serious trouble indeed. It will have to find some way to survive ... leading to the other subconscious diagnoses.

2. The Identity Problem or IDP

Love is the essential element - a universal need. Cardinal Basil Hume, head of the Catholic Church in England made the following statement in a BBC interview in the early 1990s: "Every time I conduct a marriage service, every time I see people married, I say 'that could have been me'. Deep down we remain human, very human, and we all have desires to love and to be loved by one other person."

The IDP involves a person's concept of his or her lovability, the acceptance and belonging, the rightness of his or her existence, primarily with the mother, father and even other individuals such as grandparents. I have had several patients aware, in a regression to the womb, that their mother's parents rejected the pregnancy and their daughter's involvement with the father. Sometimes it is the father's parents who reject the daughter-in-law and by implication, the baby becomes uncertain of its place in the family, the world and the universe and thus the IDP has everything to do with spiritual survival. We all have a concern about our continuance after death even if we cognitively deny it. Some of the fear associated with the concept of death has to do with this doubt of our inherent belonging - to 'not belong', to not have love, is the most powerful separation anxiety that there is. We shall talk more of this when we discuss the Death Expectancy Syndrome but it is necessary to first broaden our horizons about love itself.

In psychology and more pertinently in clinical hypnosis, the origin of the Separation Anxiety Syndrome is most often considered only in the context of the universally experienced physical separation of the baby from its mother at the moment of birth. This may be perceived by the baby as a catastrophic experience and it is of great importance. How common and damaging this is will be evident to the reader in the case discussions. However, what is not often recognised and therefore not managed in standard therapy is the fact that separation from love very often occurs *in utero*. These individuals are more vulnerable to the effects of postpartum separation.

Later separations occur in life - for example, the first day at nursery school, divorce, the termination of a relationship, the death of a loved one, geographical separation, etc. More subtle separations can occur as perceived in rejection, by not living up to the expectations of others, or in a marital argument.

The essential concept to grasp is that the loss of love, or a perception of the loss of love, is a threat to spiritual survival. To define love is not easy - there are many approaches, most of them romantic. However, the nature of love has everything to do with spiritual energy and we need to examine some aspects of it for a deeper understanding.

Spiritual survival is the subconscious mind's highest priority – one's sense of love, self, God and soul - a continuation of the spirit. Most patients we see have a narrow, limited perspective of God which is presented to them as young suggestible children in religious instruction - the theological perspective of God. This teaching has some very positive effects. It has resulted in an ordered, civilised society, and ethical and moral behaviour. It has ensured the survival of the individual, the group and belief systems.

However, there have been negative effects of this teaching in some individuals, which we will examine much more fully in discussion of the Jurisdictional Problem of Guilt. In the meantime, these negative effects include the concept of a vengeful God with potential rejection, hell and purgatory, guilt and fear.

There is another approach to God which is more philosophical and far less restrictive or manipulative. To elaborate on concepts from the last chapter, God can be described in terms of energy, thought, purpose and love.

Ritzman pointed out that the one thing we can be sure of in the universe is energy, which is the first attribute of God and which is wholly compatible with theology. In Genesis it is written: "Let there be light, and there was light." Astrophysicists have demonstrated mathematically that the first three minutes of the known universe consisted of light - photon energy, from which everything in the universe has evolved.

We interchange with this pool of energy approximately every seven years - physiologically, we exchange every atom in our bodies with our environment.

The second attribute of God is thought - since no creative effort **can** be achieved without a prior thought. There is a majestic theme to the unfolding of the universe - a divine progressive development and evolution of energy which has resulted in the creation of life. Stephen Hawking has pointed out that the universe is so fine-tuned that had the charge on the electron been only slightly less, or greater, no life would have evolved in the universe for the simple reason that no stars would have formed!

The third attribute of God is purpose - as part of the ongoing evolutionary process. We do not pretend to know what that ultimate purpose is - nor do we need to know in our moment to moment living. The point is that we are an **integral part** of this developing energy, manifested at our level by intelligent life.

The fourth attribute of God is the manner in which the above energy, thought and purpose is manifested in each of us - **love**.

We begin to have a wider perspective of the universe, of God and love - that essential energy that is inherent in each of us from the beginning, from conception. We know today that at the moment the sperm breaches the wall of the egg that there is a flash of light! Wow!!

This is the result of the release of zinc atoms. Furthermore in choosing a fertilized egg for in vitro fertilisation the egg that has the brightest flash of light carries a far better prognosis for a pregnancy. Yes there is a chemical basis for the light ... but my patients experience something much more spiritually intense.

Let us return then to the womb environment. Should anything occur which negates this love energy, it is bound to affect an individual's ability to generate and provide love and to have a negative effect on that individual's ability and potential to live life as was intended.

The mother may have many reasons for not wanting to be pregnant – she may have financial problems, she may not want to be married, she may not be married, it may interfere with a career, she may be physically ill with a serious disease, she may just be aware that emotionally she is not ready to be a mother ... or for any other reason. The result is a lessening of or absence of love ... and this is the key word, the key emotion with regard to the baby. The absence of love threatens the baby's spiritual existence. It may begin to doubt its inherent value as a creation of this universe - which it is. It is not the mother who decides which egg shall mature nor the father who decides which sperm shall fertilise that specific egg. These concepts are beyond the parents ... they belong to a vaster realm ... and they are not random selections. They are part of the unfolding, organised universal energy, a life force, a life principle ... or God. We discussed these matters in earlier chapters.

Not every baby will react negatively, of course. There is in many of them an inherent belief that not only will they survive, they will flourish. When asked where this belief, comes from a patient will usually say "from inside me." As my wife has reminded me, "not every institutionalised child becomes a psychopath!"

Occasionally, a sexual identity problem may arise from the PNE - if a baby's perception is that mother wants a boy and that being a girl will negate her acceptance and love, she may strive to be what she is not. I had a patient in just such a position and her physical appearance as an adult was that of a very hirsute - hairy - stocky woman. This patient was extremely angry with her mother for not letting her be 'me' ... repeatedly in one regression she hammered at the arm of the chair saying "why won't she let me be me?!"

3. The Death Expectancy Syndrome or DES

> *The wild hound, Fear, black, ravenous and gaunt.*
> **Lascelles Abercrombie;**
> ***Collected poems, Marriage shy. 1930.***

Fear. Fear of death ... death expectation. **All** anxiety originates in this fear, which usually begins in the birth canal where a baby feels it is in a life or death struggle but may begin in utero. This, as Dr Thomas Ritzman has said, is a universal experience for everyone delivered vaginally, at least.

Geraldine Lux Flanagan writes in her most beautiful and fairly accurate book *Beginning Life:* "Birth can be an exciting experience for the baby". This is a wholly romantic statement - and though she adds that "it is arduous", she probably has very little insight into the baby's physical and emotional confrontation with death. The baby does not **know** he or she **will** survive - its perceptions are that of tremendous pressure on its head, neck, shoulders, chest and so on. No wonder so many people experience headaches and sore necks and shoulders when they are 'under pressure'. The baby is locked into this tight canal, feels it is not progressing, begins to think 'I must breathe!' and cannot. Its arms are locked against its sides - it is helpless. During a contraction, less blood and oxygen arrives via the umbilical cord. Adrenalin - or in the USA, epinephrine, pours into its blood stream, empowering the physical body while noradrenalin hones the mind and associative thinking. Muscles tense, the heart rate accelerates dramatically. It is engulfed with a compulsion to **get out** ... or die. Small wonder we speak of 'the light at the end of the tunnel'! Anger intervenes to energise this survival. The baby struggles in vain, becomes tired ... and may give up hope.

Imagine a hunter from thirty thousand years ago - primitive man, out on the plains of Africa looking for food for himself and his family. His only weapon is a crude spear fashioned from a branch of a tree, to which he has fixed a sharp stone. He emerges from behind some rocks and suddenly, there in front of him, is a huge, hungry and mean-looking sabre-tooth tiger. Before he can react consciously, his subconscious is already at work. Adrenalin is pumped into his bloodstream. If he had time to sit back and reflect on his situation, he would notice the vigorous, rapid pumping of his heart. He would be aware that he is breathing more quickly, and perhaps taking huge gulps of air and oxygen into his lungs, to pass from there into his blood. His muscles are all tense, like a crossbow string wound up to maximum, all that potential energy waiting to be released. The pupils of his eyes are dilated - his subconscious is creating the conditions in which he can gain maximum visual information about his immediate environment. His hearing is acute ... everything is working with one goal in mind - **survival.** His subconscious knows that to survive this threat, he can do only one of two things: he must fight and kill the sabre-tooth, or he must run and escape it. This is the essence of the flight or fight response. This is the essence of fear - a survival response in the face of an actual threat, the same response a baby experiences in the birth canal. The baby's limited degree of logic is unusable because he is focussed on an immediate threat. Nobody has told him he will survive, and even if they had, his situation doesn't lend itself to sitting back and relaxing ... he has an all-encompassing biochemical and instinctual response which compels him to act ... and survive.

Once born, the baby does not have the ability to realise that he **has** survived and may already have accepted death. He may be confronted by other threats most especially the separation from the one thing that can reassure him ... mother's love. This old memory of fear therefore remains and later in life when he is confronted by other perceived threats, he will tend to react with the same feelings and thoughts. The later 'threats' may not be **real** at all ... what threat to survival can there be in a suburban supermarket? Yet our patient begins to feel claustrophobic - closed in - he starts to hyperventilate as his panic attack begins. His hyperventilation is 'merely' his subconscious response learned in the birth canal – desperate to breathe!

So **anxiety** is the same response as the fear response. The difference is that in anxiety, there is no actual immediate threat. Usually, when a threat has come and gone, we can forget it, and relax ... the adrenalin surge wanes, the heart rate returns to normal and our muscles relax. However, if we don't yet know that the threat **is** over we maintain this compulsion ... and since there is nothing to escape from, we continue to try and escape from it, maintaining a higher level of stress hormones. Anxiety, in other words, is a low-grade chronic fear in the absence of any real danger and the patient, knowing this, feels 'silly and stupid'. He is not. He just does not know **why** he is frightened. He has yet to realise that his subconscious is trying to assist him survive a threat that is long past and really irrelevant.

Of interest to me was a paper presented at the 1996 Congress of the Society of Psychiatrists of South Africa, titled *'False suffocation alarms. Spontaneous panics and related conditions: an integrative hypothesis.'* In this paper the American author hypothesises that in conditions such as panic disorder there is a physiological misinterpretation by a 'suffocation monitor' in the brain, resulting from a hypersensitivity to the level of carbon dioxide in the body. It is suggested that this misinterpretation triggers the panic reaction. This is a good example of science trying to explain a symptom on Newtonian objective grounds. It ignores the fact that this hypersensitivity is the direct result of a maximally threatening emotional memory, that the panic response is engineered by the subconscious in an effort to survive what is perceived as another threat to survival in the present, but in the absence of a real threat. The threat is a perceived one.

Most often the ISE of the Death Expectancy Syndrome is the birth process, but it may occur in the womb. If the mother is involved in an accident, or is assaulted, particularly by blows to the pregnant abdomen, the baby will experience a direct threat to survival and initiate the fear response. A threatened miscarriage similarly creates fear.

Babies born by Caesarian section do not escape the experience either. Firstly, one must consider the reason for the operation – if for an obstructed labour, the DES has already been established. If it were for toxaemia of pregnancy, a real threat exists. However, let's consider a routine, planned Caesarian section on a mother who is not in labour. As the mother is anaesthetised, the baby may report (in regression) "My mother's gone!" with immediate fear for its own survival. There is also the precipitous removal of the baby, by strong hands and fundal pressure, from the safe confines of the womb where it has been warm and loved for many months. It is suddenly taken into a much harsher environment. It is colder, it is flooded with light and much more noise, it is being handled by strangers, and worst of all it is **removed from** the mother! All these factors are threatening.

A baby is especially vulnerable to cold - its surface area:mass ratio is greater than at any other time in life and a cold environment can certainly lead to death by exposure as its body temperature drops. This is the reason why Caesarian section theatres are **warmed** to the discomfort of doctors and nurses. Indeed, if the operating room staff members are not uncomfortable, the temperature is too low.

Most of all, separation from the mother results in a disconnection of love and is termed the Separation Anxiety Syndrome, a component of the DES. It is this love which reassures the baby that it is safe, and that it can now survive. This is why 'Lamaze' babies are usually so content - they stay **with** mum, floating in the warm water and still **connected**. Separation from love is a real perceived threat to the baby's survival. This accumulates if the baby is removed to an incubator, or even to another room - the nursery. A patient will report at this moment in a regression that without this love, it cannot survive. It is without hope and helpless. Occasionally the perception is "she doesn't want me - I must be bad." A delay in feeding, or any problem with feeding, is similarly threatening.

If there has been inconsistent love within the uterus, such a person may now become very vulnerable to losing love or being separated from love in the future ... indeed, together with the IDP, the person may become a so-called 'love-addict' - dependent on outside love for his or her survival. Substitutes for love addiction include obesity, drug abuse, alcoholism, even smoking. The IDP is not the only cause of these, but certainly may be.

It is my very strong impression that 'difficult' babies such as the colicky ones, who repeatedly wake up crying, or the fretful ones, who always seem to be ill, are the result of the PNE, IDP and DES. The infant who wakes up in the middle of the night and is clearly not hungry, can be drawing attention to only two things - some pain or discomfort like a wet nappy, or fear. He or she is afraid because the traumatic physical and emotional experiences of the womb and/or birth have not been resolved ... the baby is crying for someone to tell him "it's OK, you are safe now. You are **loved and loveable**." A parent who understands this will comfort and hug the child, spend time with him until he is reminded that he is safe. A night light will be left burning in his room.

A parent who does not understand this will become concerned about his or her capabilities as a parent and may become anxious, depressed and far worse, may become angry. How will the baby respond? These things tell the baby: "it is **not** safe here. I depend on these persons for my very survival and **it is not safe**. I am **scared**, even terrified. There is **no** love. There is no hope. The only ways I can survive is by becoming very quiet and compliant, or get angry myself." Such a parent is likely to close the bedroom door and let the child 'cry himself to sleep'. What the child is doing as his cries slowly change from terror ... to anger ... and finally to the whimpering of the surrender of hope, is to accept the inevitability of his own spiritual and emotional death, his utter loneliness in a hostile world which has no understanding of his desperation.

Oh yes, he may become compliant ... the parents and their advisors will congratulate themselves on the transformation of this 'brat' into a 'good baby'. The reality of many 'good babies' is the development of a far from ideal personality, whereas the genuine good baby is the product of unconditional love - this child has no need to perform: he is aware of the rightness of his being.

Tragically, the troublesome babies are often said to be the cause of the interpersonal problems of the parents, even the cause of divorce. Would that babies could organise themselves as well as the women's liberation movements so popular in the sixties and seventies - or any other liberation movement for that matter. Oh dear me, I believe we would see an entirely different, more militant, picture. Justly so.

4. The Walking Zombie Syndrome or WZS

> *Death is all in the mind, really. Once you're dead you forget all about it.*
>
> **Jack Trevor Storey; ITV,
> Jack on the Box, 1979**

The term 'zombie' originated in Haiti. The voodoo priest, having selected his intended victim, contrives to poison him with a toxin derived from the mucus of a certain frog's skin or the blowfish. It results in a very deep coma with a cold skin, unresponsive pupils, almost indiscernible breathing and a **very** weak pulse. Not surprisingly, the victim is often declared dead and is duly buried, only to be dug up by the witchdoctor and his accomplices. Those who survive have very little control over their own volition - the toxin and prolonged low oxygen levels result in a sort of automaton who is likely to do his master's bidding. He is in effect, a 'living dead' man.

In medical hypnoanalysis, a person who has accepted his own death in some life-threatening situation, or has concluded that life is no longer worth living, becomes a 'walking zombie.' In our example in the Death Expectancy Syndrome we described a hunter confronted with a sabretooth tiger. If his flight or fight response, or anger did not provide survival, he can react in only one other way: accept his own death - **before** it has actually occurred! A true victim of the WZS commonly wears dark or black clothes, has the fixed facial features of doom and gloom and generally very little energy or enthusiasm. They sleep a lot, and get little or no satisfaction out of life. Inside, they are 'dead.'

We can 'die' at different levels, as you will remember from the order of importance. Sexual functioning is at the bottom of the list - it represents the instinctual drive to procreation and the continuation of the species. Interestingly, such are modern perceptions, when a group of **young** computer programmers was asked which level they considered to be the most important, eleven out of twelve said sexual! I'm not biased against programmers - the group essentially was young, male and so-called intelligent, certainly educated. I am pleased to report that the only one who got it right was my eldest son! All credit to him - it was with minimal direct help from me. Except that I love him.

The most obvious and easy survival threat to understand is at the physical level – for example the perception in the birth canal, when the baby has given up all hope of getting through. However, we can also die at the socio-economic level - someone who has lost his job, or has his business fail for example and is unable to provide himself or his family with the basic necessities of life, such as food and shelter. We can die at the mind level - self-esteem: how we see ourselves in our work, our family and community. And ultimately and most importantly, we can die at the spiritual level - as we have seen, when love is absent, it is a death-like feeling.

Dr Wayne Dyer discussed the fact that popular songs continuously bombard young people with this message. I am reminded of the group U2, who had the hit song "With or without you." The lyrics of the main thrust go something like this: "can't live with you, can't live without you." What the song is saying of course is that "I am dead either way." Whether we like it or not, such lyrics may subliminally reinforce hopelessness in a vulnerable teenager, while at the same time providing a sense of belonging. "If others feel like this, then at least I still have a chance of belonging to the human race." I would even postulate that the success of many pop songs is directly proportional to the emotions they evoke at these levels of identification.

So, we can become walking zombies at different levels, often more than one. Therefore, when a patient presents with, say, physical symptoms or at a sexual or socio-economic level, we already know he is 'dead' at either mind or spiritual levels: he can function only in the material world or at the sexual level so these are the problems which will surface. At the extreme child molesters fall into this group as do dis-social personality disorders or 'psychopaths' which will be discussed later.

If a person has accepted death in his own mind and life goes on, he will need some way of confirming that he **is** still alive. The alternative is to curl up in a ball, immobilised and unable to take part in the activities of the world. He will need some stimulation, perhaps, or something in his life which tells him: "hey, it's OK. I'm still here. I'm alive." A classic example is that of the post-traumatic headache - the person who has survived the coma following his car accident and head injury but has continuing, devastating headaches thereafter. The dynamics are quite straight-forward in medical hypnoanalysis.

Let us imagine someone about to be involved in a car accident. He is driving his car when he suddenly realises that there is another car coming straight at him on the wrong side of the road. He knows that it is too late to take avoiding action and a moment before the impact has the thought "Oh, oh! This is it - I'm going to die!" The cars collide, our patient has his head smashed against the windscreen or whatever and unconsciousness, a coma, ensues. His subconscious mind records this event as dying. However, he wakes up four days later and the first thing he is aware of is ...? "My head is so **sore**! ... Hang on, if I am feeling this pain then I must be alive! So as long as I feel a headache, I shall know I **am alive**!" Thus, many patients with chronic pain have their symptoms as their *proof of life* as the result of the Walking Zombie Syndrome.

CHAPTER SEVEN

More on Diagnosis

5. The Jurisdictional Problem or JDP

Every man, either to his terror or consolation, has some sense of Religion.
        James Harrington, 17th Century.

Giving every man a vote has no more made men wise and free than Christianity has made them good.
        HL Mencken

I would like to make it clear that some of the views expressed here by me are not neccessarily those of medical hypnoanalysis and may be considered controversial in some quarters. As such, they are based on my own personal experiences and from treating many patients with the JDP. Let me add that I am decidedly **not** anti-religion, just certain aspects of it.

 The JDP is a problem of guilt, where the judgement is made by the patient himself - not by God, nor necessarily by his family or community. He has taken the responsibility of jurisprudence upon himself, acting as prosecutor, judge, jury and executioner. This is based on faulty ideas and concepts and often, on perceptions of religious beliefs and doctrine: fixed concepts of heaven or hell, founded on Old Testament litany. It may arise because of confusion between the law of God and the law of man. It may arise because of confusion between the sin ... and the sinner; and it may arise when one assumes the sins of the parents.

These concepts are of course laid down early in life and act as post-hypnotic suggestions - for example, to go against the commandment 'honour thy father and mother' is to invite eternal damnation. In reality, though, there are some parents whom the child may find it very difficult to honour. Understand, yes. Forgive, hopefully – indeed necessarily. But honour? The child has not the maturity to understand, to separate the parent's behaviour from his own reactions and inherent primal purity, or to realise that the parent's behaviour is the direct result of his or her own upbringing.

What is a vulnerable child to do when endlessly confronted with tyrannical or more subtly unloving parents? Furthermore, Calvinist beliefs determine that the display of love, even within the family, is a sign of weakness. The child cannot blame the parents - from as early as the prenatal experience, he may already consider **himself** to be the 'wrong' party because he has no choice but to accept that they hold the key to his survival - he is totally dependent on them. As he grows, he cannot with impunity transgress the Ten Commandments. He must honour his mother and father. He has to find himself guilty or 'wrong' ... and does so, very often.

One must distinguish between 'shame' and 'guilt'. Guilt follows some behaviour or action which is unacceptable to society. Shame is a feeling of 'I am wrong.' As Dr RD Laing wrote in his book *Knots* published by Penguin:

> *My mother does not love me.*
> *I feel bad.*
> *I feel bad because she does not love me.*
> *I am bad because I feel bad.*
> *I feel bad because I am bad.*
> *I am bad because she does not love me.*
> *She does not love me because I am bad.*

One may substitute 'father' or 'parents'- even grandparents - for mother in the above. Dr Daniel Zelling described this emptiness of spirit as the 'hole in the soul.' This concept is an integral and essential part of Medical Hypnoanalysis. It is vital for the patient to recognise this hole in his soul, to understand precisely why it came about and to delete it ... the patient must be able to say 'I love me'', unconditionally, and without discomfort.

In terms of guilt, many children grow up with the belief that they were born with 'original sin'. Many a Christian patient whom I have treated has told me that "to be Christian is to be a sinner." That is what they are taught, either directly or by inference. This is their **perception**. Jewish patients have told me that they are not brought up to fear God, yet they are fearful. Subtly, perhaps ... subconsciously, perhaps. Psalms One and Fifteen are typical of these messages - both of which are a part of for example, the service held for the unveiling of the tombstone for a loved one passed on.

Extracts from Psalm One, verses four, five and six read: 'The ungodly are not so: but are like the chaff which the wind driveth away. Therefore the ungodly shall not stand in judgement, nor sinners in the congregation of the righteous. For the Lord knoweth the way of the righteous: but the way of the ungodly shall perish'. Psalm Fifteen, a psalm of David, asks of the Lord 'who shall abide in thy tabernacle?' and in verse four, says 'but he honoureth them that **fear** the Lord'.

Over and above the psalms and the Ten Commandments, Jewish children are given a list of six hundred and thirteen religious laws – 'mitzvot' or good deeds. These are sometimes taught as the strands of a spider's web ... with the spider sitting in the middle, of course ... waiting. I believe that anybody who can live within all these confinements is not human any longer. He is as God Himself. Yes, we are here in part, at least, to aspire to a higher spiritual level and these six hundred and thirteen laws are a positive guide in that direction. However, should a child not see the wood for the trees and take them as absolute, he may be in deep, deep trouble. Sometimes, these faulty perceptions of the mitzvot and the Commandments are the basis for severe obsessional disorders ... and psychosis. That may be an uncomfortable recognition yet it is the truth.

The intent of ancient civilisations and later religion was, I believe, to respect and actualise the Life Principle - to guide a congregation or community in terms of what society considers right and wrong; to ensure the survival of the individual as well as the group; to maximise the chances of the continuation of the race; to establish an ordered, stable civilisation. All of this is of the highest order, noble and right. It establishes the concept of conscience. We owe organised religion a great deal and shall continue to rely upon such substantial belief systems lest civilisation deteriorates into primitive barbarism. Unfortunately, despite religion, many so-called civilised areas of the world have already done so. Sometimes this is written into secular law – South Africa's constitution keeps a murderer from the hangman, yet sanctions the elimination of utterly defenceless sentient babies through abortion. Radical belief systems serve their own selfish purpose.

The route chosen to achieve this advancement of humanity was through the medium of fear. Fear of divine punishment ... through guilt. This holds true for ancient spiritual beliefs as well - be they worshippers of the sun or Zeus or ancestors. It is possible that some more recent religions have lost their way, and are out of touch with the reality of modern times, just as we consider ancient beliefs to be. Who is to judge beliefs - do they not largely achieve the same purpose? I find it difficult to accept that God told man (Jews and Moslems at least) to forever abstain from pork - with the penalty of risking damnation to hell or rejection by their deity. Years ago, the educated clergy were well aware that pork was infested with parasites ... were they not advising an uneducated and ignorant group in their best interests, with the best of motives?

I have no problem speaking from my own experience. As a nine year old I was given the privilege of carrying the Torah from the Ark to the pulpit, or the 'bimah'. I had of course been warned by my well-meaning friends that the Torah was really heavy. Walking towards the Ark, the cantor warned me: "If you let the Torah fall, everyone in shul will have to fast for forty days and forty nights!" What a senseless thing to say to a child. What negativity. What **fear**. What manipulation. He could just as easily have said that the Torah was light - which it was, even to a nine year old. He could just as easily have been encouraging and advised he'd be with me to assist if I ran into problems - which he was. The result of my experience was to determine that not all religious people were as gentle and loving as my revered Rabbi was. I became wary. Very wary. And afraid.

The following is a short extract from one of my patients, whom, when asked in the history if she had ever feared God, replied: "Terrified, still am!" Let us consider a pertinent regression of hers - she was asked to go back to the time that her fear of God arose: her responses were clipped and filled with angst.

T	: How old are you?
Gina	: Five.
T	: What is happening?
Gina	: Nun. With a big stick. Going to smack me.
T	: For what reason?
Gina	: Because I'm bad.
T	: What have you done, Gina?
Gina	: Don't know what I've done. Afraid! Must come up and be smacked. I don't understand.
T	: How much power does she have, Gina?
Gina	: All! She's God's bride!
T	: Who told you that, Gina?
Gina	: The nuns told me.
T	: If she's cross, what does that mean to you?
Gina	: Pain! God's cross. God is not nice. I don't care!!

Her confrontation with what she perceived as God's direct messengers was not over - at seven years of age she experienced an intensifying event. Our patient Gina was informed by the priest of the following - and note, they may not have been his direct words, but they were certainly her **perception**:

"You must be good like Jesus, but if you recognise yourself as good, that is pride, and pride is **bad**. You must be like Jesus but you can't be because you are not a man."

She received the powerful impression that "Women are evil! Women must do what men want!" We are talking here of a small girl, who could not use logic and who found it a sin to question what she was told - she held this idea into her forties, until in hypnosis we were able to remove her faulty beliefs. We are also locked in, with these statements, with the culture of two thousand years ago when women had no real status ... this **was** the *status quo* of the time.

According to a Christian radio sermon I recently heard, to join God's family one **has** to embrace Jesus Christ. In the first place this ignores the reality that at conception we are inherently a part of God's family. In the second place, this sermon by all logic is patently absurd, as it excludes the bulk of the human race! Jesus is of course one pathway to God, but there are many wholesome pathways.

What is a child to do in these circumstances? What this patient did was to cease going to church. She had lived in fear of God's judgement and punishment ever since. She found herself guilty and unworthy. Now, that particular nun clearly had a problem - and as adults we can understand that - she was after all a human being and we are nowhere near perfect. However, her pupil's perceptions of God, together with her home life, resulted in a disaster. The priest...? Well, the less said of him, the better. Or perhaps he was misunderstood.

The Catholic intervention of Mother Mary on behalf of women certainly helped her, but did not eradicate her fear of not being good enough for Jesus, of not being accepted by God. It is this fear which determines how destructive the guilt will be ... punishment is a sequel to guilt and this self-imposed punishment is damaging to that person's life ... perhaps as minimally as a migraine, but sometimes as life-threatening as in some cancers, or becoming totally dissociated from the mainstream of life as in psychosis.

Another less physically damaging consequence, yet just as catastrophic for that particular religion, is that the person alienates himself or herself from that belief system - they must do so to survive! This, I believe, is a contributor to the dilution of religious belief seen in the world today. It is a major cause of atheism and it thereafter requires a major threat - individual, national or global - for that person to return to religious faith ... to love, which is what was missing in the first place. Unfortunately, many of these people returning to religion often do so with fanatical observance, still without this love.

The truth is that, whatever colour, culture or creed, we all come from the same source of love. Again and again therapists find that the need of the majority of patients is for love. If love was not present - in fact or by perception - the thought that God 'may not love me' condemns that person to a miserable life, as his last hope is dashed. It encourages a path in life which leads to ensuring that everyone around him is happy while denying his own needs. Why? Because such a person is compelled to ensure no further loss of love ... this would be catastrophic - spiritual death. Those who find that even this behaviour achieves little may well exclude all guilt and responsibility as threatening ... and become Conduct Disorders, Dissocial Personalities or psychopaths.

Let us take sex as another example. The forbidding of masturbation and to 'spill seed', or to make love to one's wife except for limited times of her menstrual cycle is clearly a manoeuvre which will increase the chances of impregnation and survival of the race. I do not believe that these laws follow the life principle. God created us with the gift of sexual pleasure - toddlers masturbate, for goodness' sake! It is an entirely natural phenomenon. Is it then to be considered a sin? Is there an arbitrary divide? Must one switch off on attaining puberty? Can one? No. Not without diminishing one's essential humanity. Onan was punished not for spilling his seed, but for disobedience. Religious doctrines have become a teaching device to inform children that public masturbation is not acceptable. Quite rightly - this has established another facet of civilised life or conscience. However, to the child caught masturbating and criticised it is the end of the world. Calvinist religions are even worse in many respects ... in terms of the twentieth century. We had a President of South Africa country who declared on national TV 'we are a God-**fearing** nation!' Aye, there's the rub.

Wars have been fought and millions have died, in the interests of religion and religious conviction. In the 1980's in the Iran/Iraq war a million young men went to do battle allegedly with the firm belief that to die would mean instant acceptance by God and entry into heaven. The current wars in Iraq further this wanton destruction of lives and historic property. Religious doctrine was the basis of the crusades centuries ago. It makes one wonder what type of people direct such catastrophes, which consume the lives of the young, the cream of the future, from both opposing factions. A private study of their behaviour convinces me that many of them are dissocial personality disorders - psychopaths. There are many examples of such tyrants - Hitler, Stalin, Idi Amin, Genghis Khan. Some people disagree with me when I include Alexander the Great. By and large, their followers will obey orders because they fear not only immediate retribution by the society of the time ... but also divine retribution. Such is the history of Mankind.

A principle of Christianity is that man is a fallen spirit. "You were born with original sin!" It was David who said this, not God. How long must humankind endure the failings of Adam and Eve? The sins of the father passing endlessly down, generation after generation, eon after eon. The ministry of religious affairs in Israel reportedly maintained a list of people who are banned from marriage because they are classed as 'bastards' or 'impure'. One report was of a woman refused permission to marry because one of her ancestors 2500 years ago, a priest, had married a divorcee - breaking a religious law. The law was then imposed on all his descendants. Another example: a child resulting from a woman's affair or rape is considered a bastard and so are all the progeny for the next ten generations! Assuming the sins of the parent, indeed! Labelled.

I reject this concept. We cannot live in fear, not without sacrificing our God-given humanity and lessening our ability to generate, magnify and give love: which is essentially our duty, our purpose and greatest pleasure on earth.

Most children **have** already masturbated before being warned of transgressing these laws on penalty of damnation - masturbation is an entirely normal feature of human development! Laws forbidding masturbation were designed to maximise the chances of conception, ensuring the continuation and survival of the race. These children, if vulnerable, cannot confess their 'already committed' sins - though Catholicism and other religions conveniently provide for this. Children are loathe to discuss their sexual feelings and actions for fear of the reaction - which they see as potential rejection or as not honouring their mother and father.

Quoting from an article in a Jewish newspaper, the Talmud according to scholars, finds that the Jewish Day of Atonement 'atones for the sins between human beings and God, but not for sins between human beings. You can only right these wrongs in one of two ways - firstly to seek forgiveness from whom you have wronged. Secondly, there must be a change in behaviour.'

The latter is absolutely true. However, changing behaviour presents a major obstacle because it is based on survival responses as a result of an unavailable subconscious memory. Yes, it can be done by a sustained effort of conscious will. Yet, ultimately the subconscious will triumph in its endeavour to survive ... in imprinted subconscious ways which are beyond the conscious mind's ability to control. So while a wayward husband may indeed try successfully to make amends to his wife and be faithful, should his perceived survival threat again become strong enough, more often than not his old behaviour will be repeated.

Atonement is a tricky concept. Certain religious beliefs and philosophies utilise denial quite openly as a protection. For example "True denial is a powerful protective device. You can and should deny any belief that error can hurt you. This kind of denial is not a concealment but a correction."

Herein lies an incongruency - something is not ringing true - because this particular belief system holds that "therefore denial is not used to hide anything, but to correct error."

The key word is **error**. 'Error' is the 'evil' so many religious doctrines collude with. 'Error' is the deviation from perfection and anything 'less than perfect is not of God'. Thus the person committing the error is evil. This twisted logic is the cause of great suffering - an 'evil' in itself.

In the first place, we are not created 'perfect'. Humans are imperfect in that we are created with enormous potential but are entirely vulnerable and impressionable. Were there ever to be a 'perfect' human, that person would be as God himself – God in the purely theological sense. I would think that this imperfection is part of our drive to improve our inner selves, to reach higher levels of spirituality. The point is, imperfection is inherent in us and is reduced by positive learning. The universe itself is imperfect - it is violent! Natural disasters occur on a scale unimaginable by most people. Our own Milky Way is slowly attracting smaller satellite galaxies with its huge gravitational effect, eg the Magellan and Sagittarius galaxies: imagine two galaxies colliding!! How can we then presume to be perfect? Interestingly, such a collision and events like supernovae allowed us to evolve - it resulted in the heavier elements essential to life.

In the second place, atonement as prescribed by theology is based on love - the loving acceptance of God. The tragedy is that many of the people I see sought this atonement because of their inherent **fear** of God. It is here that a critical divergence occurs. Fear is one of the weapons which maintains civilisation. If this primary fear were not present, no atonement would be needed but civilisation would be vulnerable. One answer is to recognise the difference between 'conscience' and 'guilt', conscience being that behaviour which is acceptable to society. A second route is to eliminate the fear of God and the subsequent guilt with its self-imposed punishment, for to the subconscious it is better to suffer in this life rather than for all eternity. To do this requires the 'simple' acceptance of oneself as an inherent part of the universe and its energy - **ab initio**!

This energy is love, and love is God. 'Error' is the result of the absence of love. In the absence of love there is fear ... and guilt. In some important ways formal theology has contributed to guilt, perpetuated guilt and intensified guilt - while at the same time perpetuating atonement and an endless loop of problems.

Thirdly, the truth is that **all** 'error' is the result of attempts to survive at one or other level on the order of importance. This survival is an instinctual, inherent ... and if you like, a God-given compulsion. If one has subconsciously accepted death at the spiritual and mind levels, there will be a need to find some way of knowing 'I am still alive' at a lower level - physical or territorial or sexual. 'Territorial' naturally includes one's socio-economic status - material things. Behaviour such as habitual stealing is a proof of life at this level because these people are mind and spiritually dead.

Stealing is of course unacceptable behaviour to society - this is an 'error'. However, in a child who is always stealing his classmates' property or is otherwise destructive, the true dynamics are instinctual compulsions of survival. All so-called 'error' **can** be explained ... there **is** a reason for each one. And it is one's learned experiences which determine each one.

No fetus in the womb has committed an 'error' - the moment of his or her conception is the expression of creative love ... and that energy **is** God. There is an inherent peace in this newly created life at this time but the fetus is like a blank sheet cognitively or intellectually ... like an incredibly sophisticated computer with an enormous capacity for recording data. The quality of the imprinted data - the suggestions accepted or the programming - will determine exactly how that computer responds later on in accordance with its preprinted circuit boards - or genetic code.

The vulnerable child absorbs information - by autosuggestion and that provided from outside - as time passes. Its programming will determine its future thoughts, feelings and behaviour. These reactions are and will be modified by its genetic component and further experiences.

Society dictates that atonement must come in one way or another - and it is usually in the form of self-judgment and self-punishment, which is a major cause of human misery - from cancer in some cases, to obsessive-compulsive disorders, from anorexia/bulimia to migraine to… Many of my patients had this guilt and separation from God as the core of their disorder. How much healthier and happier to accept a God who loves, who understands and forgives without the trappings of arbitrary man-made laws. Perhaps mankind is not yet ready for this ... or is he? The way that 'civilisation' is heading, man had better be ready ...

A danger of the atonement principle is that if a person's perception is that he has **not** experienced forgiveness, or has not experienced some sudden spiritual belonging, his negative beliefs may be reinforced. And even with forgiveness, should his 'error' behaviour recur, he is confused.

All these vectors - of the judgement of religion, the judgement of society, his family - increase his negativity until he judges himself.

In the worst possible scenario, he has less and less hope of forgiveness, dies more and more at spiritual and mind levels and ultimately says "screw the world and God". Free now from guilt he becomes a dissocial personality disorder, or 'psychopath' and his behaviour becomes less and less acceptable to society - a vicious cycle indeed.

Interestingly, history records that when mankind has been confronted with devastation, he turns in great numbers to God. However, present statistics show that attendances at synagogues are down in many areas, as are attendances at church. The number of nuns has declined to almost crisis levels, even the number of priests.

Intermarriage, once - and still - considered a most terrible sin or 'error', is on the increase. Why should this be happening? Could it be that in their endeavour to hold on to the flock, religion has created the rigid conditions that encourage a dispersion? Every atheist I have treated chose this way of life to avoid divine punishment. Sometimes it was a conscious decision, most often it was subconscious. Interesting ... in their history they consciously declared they did not believe in God ... yet, in hypnosis declared their fear of Him.

Religion is unfortunately also used by many people to justify their anger. Sometimes God is used as the scapegoat - particularly when a person's rotten experiences in life seem to contradict everything he was taught about Him - that He is always there. In therapy, many patients verbalise something like this: "Well, what about the children who were born as Down's Syndrome and so on? What reason would God have for such a tragedy?" Most of these people are trying to rationalise life in terms of what they were taught and the reality of life as they have experienced it. However, there are observations to be made here. Firstly, these people are clinging to the image of childhood where they see God as a person, only infinitely more powerful - and that **he controls** them. They have not matured sufficiently to realise that God **is** the universe, love and probably more; that He has created the conditions for us to grow, but that it is **our** responsibility to use these opportunities; that the universe is an uncertain place. Secondly in this vein and I again quote

Dr Bernie Siegel: "Most of us want God to change the external aspects of our lives so we don't have to change internally. We want to be exempt from the responsibility for our own happiness".

I am aware that these statements of mine will probably result in a furore of protest and I shall likely be branded, at least metaphorically, as a heretic or worse. The truth is that I am more spiritual today than I have ever been; that I am closer and more at peace with the creator than at any time in my past, and that I utilise my patients' religious convictions in a positive manner to reinforce their own belief and faith and occasionally to re-establish it! The very nature of this work is centred on the reality of man's role as part of His universe.

What I am emphasising is that while religion plays an essential, positive role in the development of man, there are certain individuals who are susceptible to its potential negative effects - who largely present with severe emotional and physical distress based on fear and guilt. It may be that in religion's altruism, it has been hoist by its own petard or injured by its double-edged sword of guilt. I am not convinced that organised religion recognises this to the extent that it can provide effective counselling to some people, who see this as contradictory. Clearly, these patients, treated by myself and many others, have not experienced significant assistance from their respective religious bodies. One wonders if the time has not come to educate children with a different perspective of the Ten Commandments.

Quote:

> *I can hardly think that there was ever any scared into Heaven.*
> **Sir Thomas Browne. 17th Century.**
> **Religio Medici.**

6. The Ponce de Leon Syndrome or PDL

> *Nothing would induce me to go over my childhood days again.*
> *I thought I was happy because my mother said I was.*
> **Rev HRL Sheppard;** Quoted
> Carolyn Scott, Dick Sheppard

Ponce de Leon was the governor of Puerto Rico more than five centuries ago - it was he who was told by one of the islanders that the now fabled 'fountain of youth' lay on one of the nearby islands, and that to bathe in its waters would arrest the ageing process. Ponce de Leon was not that keen on getting old after his retirement and determined to find this fountain. He organised two expeditions to that end - paid for, by the way, by the king of Spain. He never found it of course…

The Ponce de Leon syndrome describes the problem of emotional immaturity. On the basis of a now established identity problem, or the WZS or DES etc, we may become arrested in our emotional development as we grow through childhood. A very common example of this is a child caught masturbating and subsequently castigated by a parent. 'That is evil. You must not do that again.' You may laugh at this archaic approach but believe me it occurs commonly in the late twentieth century - with devastating effects.

The child's train of thought is now: 'My mother or my father rejects this. There is a lessening of love. That is threatening to me. It felt pleasureable but it is wrong. I must be wrong. I will go to the devil if I do it again. God rejects me. I will not do it again.' Sometimes the thought is 'sexual pleasure is wrong!' and this often results in masochistic sexual practice – 'I must feel pain to enjoy sex'!

When the child, say a girl, now reaches puberty she is reminded of a negative sexual connotation, that she is being evil by simply becoming a woman. She is scared (DES) to say anything and feels guilty (JDP). She must punish herself … and what better way than to have **pain** with this 'awful' admission of womanhood. She develops dysmenorrhoea - period pain. She may view sex as something evil and necessary only for procreation. No pleasure! A duty.

She becomes locked into this immature reaction of thinking, feeling and behaving … to allow herself pleasure or a pain-free period is to her subconscious to invite death at the spiritual level. She cannot progress because of the fear of faulty beliefs established by her perceptions from an ignorant parent when she was perhaps three or four years old.

A multitude of other problems may arise because of similar post-hypnotic suggestions given in childhood, some of which we will discover in the case discussions. The crux is that to grow older than that particular age is dangerous to that individual - either at a physical, self-worth or spiritual level. Our task is to remove the fear of growing older and the need the patient had at the time of his or her maturation arrest: this need was usually love.

* * *

The **Examination** of the Patient: **The Word Association**

Imagine that we now have taken the history and have a good idea of what the critical events were - we have a presumptive subconscious diagnosis. The next stage of medical hypnoanalysis, following the medical model, is to **examine** the patient and confirm the diagnoses and events. As any good teacher of medicine will tell you, the diagnosis is made on the history - the examination merely confirms it.

At this stage the medical doctor would take the patient's blood pressure, and temperature, examine the throat and listen to the heart and lungs, etc. The examination in medical hypnoanalysis consists of a **word association exercise**, or WAE - and this is undertaken **in** hypnosis. All, or certainly most of the succeeding sessions are in hypnosis - there is little point in talking to only the conscious mind as it doesn't know what the heck the real problem is. Most patients arriving for medical hypnoanalysis have already been through this already and while many say, rightfully, that they were assisted more say they felt they 'didn't get to grips with the matter.'

The WAE is of a standardised design (Dr William Bryan's great contribution, together with the concept of the Walking Zombie Syndrome) and is used by medical hypnoanalysts around the world. Naturally it allows for some prompts to be individualised to each patient. Very simply, a series of words or phrases are given to the hypnotised patient, who responds with whatever first comes into his or her mind - be it another word, phrase, place or person etc. These are recorded and later the therapist will review the responses, looking for associations which confirm already known facts and provide new insights into that particular patient. It assists in accurately identifying the really significant events that need to be looked at and worked through in therapy. This is a great time- and money-saving device because it means we do not have to dodder through a patient's entire life. The subconscious mind **knows**, so we gratefully utilise that knowledge.

If we are still not quite sure, or would like more information, we do our **investigation** - the next stage of the medical model, just as a doctor might order a throat swab, x-rays or blood tests. In medical hypnoanalysis, this is achieved with a **dream analysis** or some other hypnotic technique. The patient is given a suggestion that he will have a particular dream, one that has to do with the very origin of the problem. The subconscious mind is wonderfully symbolic and our dreams reflect what is going on - they are a direct window into the subconscious.

Many books have been written about the symbolic meaning of dreams. Freud started the rot and was heavily biased towards sexual connotations, as in the snake for example representing a phallic symbol. Dreams are highly individualised and certain symbols may have different meanings for different people. For example, one of my patients had a snake as the symbol blocking his progress. It had nothing to do with sex, at least not directly ... it had to do with ... **guilt!** It was the serpent which suggested Adam and Eve eat the forbidden apple. Now **there** was a post-hypnotic suggestion from childhood!

OK! Now, for the next stage of the therapy - the work-up has been completed and we are ready to lance the boil and release the pus. The act, in the medical model, of **healing.**

CHAPTER EIGHT

The Healing Process of Medical Hypnoanalysis

- My Own Experience

Life is like a flame that is always burning out; but it catches fire again every time a child is born.
George Bernard Shaw; The Adventures of the Black Girl in her search for God.

The healing process is easily and succinctly reduced to the seven 'Rs' as follows: The first is the 'R' of **Rapport** - this is what the therapist has been allowing and encouraging to happen when taking the history and providing an explanation of hypnosis and during the therapy. This entails the development of a mutual trust and respect, which is of the greatest importance, for without this, the process is stormy. The patient may project anger, negative emotions and other needs onto the therapist, who if he's not aware, may well send these right back to the patient. While not catastrophic, it certainly puts paid to any constructive work and leaves both parties with decidedly negative vibes.

The next 'R' is **Relaxation** - the first formal session of hypnosis where the primary objective is to help the patient experience as deep a trance as possible, while providing a series of protective suggestions and reinforcing the patient's sense of control, and cementing the rapport. There is hardly a closer therapeutic relationship than this, and this fact is openly acknowledged and appreciated - by me, anyway. The patient is now usually taught how to do self-hypnosis and given an hypnosis CD to listen to regularly.

The next 'R' is the healing process itself and consists of the tool of **Regression** in trance back to those significant events to review and change the effect they had. Thus, **Realisation** is the next 'R' - the patient is able to find out what his perceptions and beliefs were and how they affected his way of thinking, feeling and behaving. The fifth 'R' is to **Remove** those faulty beliefs and, six, **Replace** them with a positive belief. For example : 'Yes, I realise how frightened I was at six weeks of age when I fell from my mother's arms face down into the full baby bath - I was scared I would drown and die. That was a reasonable response at that age, but I know today I was not in any danger because my mother picked me up immediately and gave me love. I also realise that I **didn`t** die - I am very much alive and I don't need to be afraid of water any more. I could probably drink the whole bath tub of water today. I can even imagine myself swimming in the sea, very comfortably'.

The seventh and final 'R' is that of **Reinforcement** of the new belief and **Rehabilitation** of the old automatic negative reactions resulting ultimately in automatic positive reactions. This process, one can see, has already begun.

It **is** that 'simple'. As someone once said "I can't see why one should complicate things, if the simple idea works." Well, it does - for most people, rapidly and effectively, with long lasting results. Frankly, the failures I see are in those patients who remain afraid ... and this is often at subconscious level. As if to say, 'if I let go of my symptom I will again be in danger. I can't trust you or myself yet to let that happen.' Alternatively 'I am such a bad person I still don't deserve a happy fulfilling life.'

Interestingly, while some patients fall into this category - about fifteen percent - they sometimes come back later and are successful. The ice has been broken, some fundamental change has taken place, an idea has been planted that perhaps this **is** possible ... and when they **are** ready, they can do what is needed for themselves. The point is, **they** can do it - essentially it is the patient who does the healing. It doesn't hurt though, to have a trained and caring professional to assist!

I promised to tell my own story - how I became involved in hypnotherapy, as well as the more personal problems I encountered.

There is an answer for everything: one just has to go back far enough and find out **why** a person reacts in a way that is self destructive.

On the surface, I had a perfectly stable childhood, even privileged, though my parents were not well off and sometimes really struggled financially. Both of them worked hard for a better life for their children. I had an excellent academic record at school and was well liked by everyone. I was a leader of the student body both at primary and high school levels. I excelled in sport - rugby, cricket, swimming, field hockey and even gained junior provincial colours in the latter. I gained a commission during my compulsory military service and received the top award as the leading candidate officer in the armoured corps. At university I withdrew more into the background, while maintaining success at social, academic and sporting levels. I passed every year at medical school - which only about forty percent of the student body managed. I was commended on my performance as an intern and was encouraged by my seniors to specialise. As I was already married with a child, financial needs determined that rather than specialise I enter family practice ... and I was hugely successful.

However, I would like to correct the notion held by some people that being a GP is fairly straightforward - very busy perhaps, but not really a 'big deal'. Besides being called upon to make hundreds of critical decisions each day, there are often situations which are extremely stressful. The following are a few examples from my practice.

I was called on my pager (indicating my age!) to urgently attend a patient - the problem was not described to me but I knew she was not a patient of mine. Medical ethics demand that a doctor is obliged to provide a service in cases of emergency, so I responded to the call, knowing I still had four more visits to make before attending my packed consulting rooms, for which I was already late.

I arrived at the address, grabbed my bag from the back seat of my car and ran through the open door of the house, expecting someone to greet me with whatever problem there was. The following picture presented itself. A woman and her two young children were cowering in fear on the couch in the sitting room. I was dimly aware that there were pock marks on the wall behind them and it passed through my mind that either they were not very house proud or were having tough financial times. The reason for this scene was on my right - in my peripheral vision there was someone on my right in the middle of the room. An almost tangible aura of danger was immediately apparent, as was the pungent odour of burnt cordite.

The husband was standing there with a .38 calibre revolver in his hand and appeared quite 'over the edge'. I suddenly realised that the pock marks were the result of several rounds from that gun! This was a situation of an impending family murder ... and I was in the middle with a fair chance of becoming the first statistic!

The subconscious mind is a wonderful thing: the fight or flight response is immediately there to assist. But I could neither fight nor run away. Firstly, because he would probably shoot - his gun wavered in my direction - and secondly because for some ethical reason, I **had** to help the family, as well as myself, in self-preservation. So, with eight lectures on general psychology from my fourth year of study, I had to deal with it. My mind became as clear as crystal - ideas and their alternatives were assessed and rejected in microseconds. I decided that the route was to portray myself as totally in his power and appeal to some possible semblance of reason in this man. Actually, I **was** totally in his power - at that moment he could have chosen life or death for me.

I cannot remember what I said, but it obviously was the right stuff. After some minutes - which seemed like a lifetime - he surrendered his weapon and allowed the police to be called.

I've delivered a premature baby of a mother with encephalitis, resuscitated the baby and then repaired her episiotomy - all by torchlight and with the assistance of a male nurse who was not qualified in midwifery. I have done a tracheotomy on a baby with croup who had respiratory failure, also by torchlight! I have talked down two very aggressive schizophrenics and a young man with a drug psychosis. I have been called to deal with an adult rinkhals - a venomous snake - who did not appear to be very charmed by the interruption. During a particularly bad winter with a flu epidemic I once saw 102 patients between the hours of 5 am and 1.30 am the next morning: that didn't make me rich - the tax man took a seventy two percent cut. I worked for two weeks to cover expenses, for about ten days to pay the tax man and the balance for myself. If we took a long weekend away, there was simply no money to draw. When I left general practice for a while, all I had to show for seven years of hard work was a bank overdraft.

No-one must tell me that general practice is not stressful!

However, we all survived. So, why should this picture of success come crashing down? How did it? The truth is that in my early thirties I became addicted to pethidine - meperidine in the USA - and my entire world crashed and burned. Pethidine is a powerful synthetic narcotic. Actually, the crash and burn happened just before the addiction - the Symptom Intensifying Event.

My first wife was a very troubled person. I bear no grudges towards her and we remain on good terms. She knows I am relating this story - though the perceptions are mine. Her own history is not unlike that of many patients I have treated and the tragedy is that she was never afforded the opportunity of having her own analysis. She saw the best available professionals, who had no answers and were ethically very evasive when I asked them for a diagnosis. I have no doubt whatsoever that the course of her life - and mine - may have been very different with individual analysis. But then again, much else of my life would not have been realised! There is indeed, a reason for every speck of dust that flies. No coincidences.

As to her diagnosis - in traditional and medical hypnoanalytic terms – it is not fair to comment. Perhaps she needed a sense of freedom. Speculation, in any event, is pointless. For my part, she might well have cause to say that I worked long and hard hours. That in winter, when the whole world seemed to be ill, I would not get home at any kind of reasonable hour. My first two children used to wait up patiently to see me before going to bed, until 8 or 9 pm. Sometimes I was too late and they would be fast asleep. However, I was just doing what I had to do at that time. Problems and conflicts arose. She sought acceptance elsewhere. I now know that confrontation only served as a survival threat to her.

Eventually, she declared her love for another person to me ... and this was my own Symptom Intensifying Event, as well as hers, for the addiction. I believed that I had reached the end of my resources, was a failure, and yet I was trapped in a very powerful feeling of responsibility for her and our children. I had made certain marriage vows. Besides, here I was - the ultimate GP - with a marriage falling apart and I could do nothing about it. What an example! Unacceptable. No. There was no way to turn, no escape. My adrenalin flow heightened with this unrecognised threat of guilt ... and then ebbed. Inside, I accepted it was the end. I wasn't thinking of physical death, in fact I wasn't thinking at all. I was **feeling** spiritual death, mind death. There seemed no hope. I became a walking zombie. And she was feeling as dead as I was ... the charge of emotion had found a way through her subconscious needs, there was a realisation of the potential effects of the situation.

When a person 'dies' in one part, the rest of that person is still experiencing life but there is an uncertainty about it. Something is needed to confirm that one **is** still alive ... some stimulation, some excitement, some pain or some difficulty which will bring relief to this dilemma. When she suggested then and there that we use some pethidine, I at first rejected the idea. The consequences were unacceptable. However, the situation was overwhelming ... and so it began. The use of pethidine had two effects.

Firstly, there was the typical euphoric effect of a narcotic - a warmth and security that removed the problems of the world entirely. They were simply somewhere else ... of no consequence at all while floating somewhere in the clouds of unreal peace. So relieving of soul pain was it that the next day could be seen through ... with the promise of another escape that evening.

Secondly, more subtly and potentially far more dangerous, there was a return of the co-dependence of our relationship. The marriage survived. So the addiction we both developed was a proof of life in two ways: individually for her and me, and the marriage. Now you will say **'what?!'** Surely you knew that the addiction would doom both of you in a fairly short time? Why would you do **that?!** That's so **stupid!** Of course, you're right.

This is a very good example of the mechanisms of the subconscious mind. The reason, as we've discussed before, is that the subconscious will choose a means of survival in any situation, which even though obviously dangerous, is **less threatening** than the alternative of that moment ... and the alternative at that time for me and for her was ... death. Spiritual and mind death. Anything was better than that. And ... emotion is far more powerful and compelling than logic.

Our addiction lasted about eighteen months. The use of pethidine rose from one ampoule of 100 mg per day to fifty ampoules a day, each. Ten amps at a time, intravenously. The intervention by the police - the Narcotics Bureau - aggravated the situation: initially there was increased anxiety, then 'what the hell' – it was all out in the open anyway. The worst had happened - I was facing a sentence of twenty years in jail for dealing in drugs. So nothing mattered any more. All hope was lost and there were no further restraints.

Rather than reduce or stop the use of narcotics, the addiction very rapidly increased. We became expert at finding the tiniest veins and gaining access with a 26 gauge needle. We each endured several epileptic seizures as a result of unintentional overdoses. At the end, we would remain 'high' only for some minutes - we needed ten amps just to avoid the withdrawal, to be able to function! Sometimes, we would 'shoot' half an hour too early, overloading the reticular activating system of the brain and ... fit, have an epileptic seizure. One of these resulted in my suffering an alleged cardiac arrest, from which she says she resuscitated me. She called a friend and colleague of mine who arranged an immediate admission to a clinic and the long road to recovery began. To her credit and mine - I'm not ashamed to say so - we both survived. About twenty-five other professionals were fellow patients over the next few years ... of these, none have survived. Just we two… the others? They died from overdoses, accidents, suicides.

One of the psychiatrists who initially treated my wife was a renowned and august figure in medical and legal circles. At one stage, when we were trying to get off the habit, she was in severe withdrawal, and becoming really desperate - something which can only be appreciated by a narcotic addict. I called this colleague - her psychiatrist - for advice, assistance, admission to a clinic, anything. His advice was "Give her some grass to smoke". I was shattered. We had never smoked marijuana. I thought that if this was the best that psychiatry could offer, we had no chance at all. **Our** reaction to **his** uncaring attitude precipitated a return to, and escalation of, addiction.

It was only when we asked the late Dr Sylvain De Miranda for help that any understanding of addiction and some structure and discipline became available. My recovery was perhaps easier than hers because I was now staring physical death in the face if I continued, perhaps with the very next dose. I had no veins anyway, they were all thrombosed.

We were admitted to a clinic for withdrawal, and I remember the first few days as being horrendous, despite adequate alternative drugs. Apparently, I did not progress too well, because the next thing I remember was waking up in total darkness - as I found out, nearly three days later.

I awoke with no prior knowledge of anything - no memory, nothing. I was lying on something I eventually recognised as a bare mattress in absolute blackness. I had no idea of place or time, or even who I was. Strangely, there was no anxiety - only curiosity. I had a flashing fantasy that maybe I was a spy. Night or day? Must be night, because there was no light anywhere. Deciding I could not just lie there, I got up to explore this void, and promptly fell ... onto cold smooth concrete. Crawl, then. I crawled. One shuffle at a time, then extending my right hand forward to touch something, still not knowing who I was. I felt physically fine, there was just this blankness, and the darkness. Eventually, I touched something solid - a wall, I recognised with some excitement. I stood up slowly, let the dizziness pass and began to move to my left, right hand on the wall. One corner. Further ... another corner. A little panic - what if there were just corners? Then, something else - I recognised a door. Cold - steel. A door. My hands were all over it, exploring for a handle. I didn't find one, but did find an inset in the door - like a hatch? Did it open? I slid it to the left and light, blessed light flooded in. As I looked out I saw a courtyard unfamiliar to me ... and then all the memories flooded back. And I realised I must have been in a cell and heavily sedated. Triumphant now, exhilarated because I felt no withdrawal, I called to a couple of my fellow patients out there to summon a nurse - I was ready to rejoin the world.

I had made a **decision to live**, though I did not realise the significance of this then, nor even formulate it as such in my mind.

That was the critical moment. I decided to live not just at a physical level but at every other level. One morning I had a cathartic episode ... and it came out of the blue. I **knew** I could put the past - **all** the past - behind me, that I could be a happy and fulfilled person by choosing to be one. It was the most uplifting moment of my life. It was sheer energy and not a little faith. Sure, I still had work to do ... hypnoanalysis wasn't available then, not in South Africa.

Once the decision had been made I experienced a feeling of relief - I no longer had to hide. In fact, the more people who knew about what had happened, the better: there would be more chance of someone recognising a 'slip', a return to the addiction, and intervening.

When we did divorce about three years later, allowing her custody of my children was one of the hardest decisions of my life, for I was scared for them. At the same time I knew instinctively that if I kept them, she might run into a brick wall, she would no longer have any purpose in life. I had a gut feeling that she needed them more than I. It was less difficult to go to where they lived few years later and bring them back to stay with us - things were not ideal there. I was now married again with a new baby. But it was still difficult. Through these years, a little book called *Your Erroneous Zones* by Dr. Wayne Dyer helped, as did the dedicated professionals led by Dr Sylvain de Miranda, to whom I am eternally grateful, and my dearest friend in the world ... my wife Beverley... and the three greatest children in the universe: Steven, Melissa and Roderick. I owe so many people a great debt of gratitude - the patients of my practice and my medical colleagues, my parents and brothers and friends, who believed in me. They gave me the courage to believe in myself.

Today my first wife has achieved her own contentment and fulfilment - she has remarried and leads a productive life. She has survived, far more successfully than some would have believed possible - and all credit to her.

One thing more ... I do not recommend addiction to a narcotic as a growth experience. I will not bore you with the finer details of the tragedy, misery and pain of addiction ... I've been there, it's bad, horrendously bad ... it is now over, and has been for more than forty years. Believe me, there are easier ways to find a new road in life.

Let's look at why and how it all happened - how I became a Prisoner of my Own Perceptions. 'Pooped'.

Imagine a baby ... a baby floating in a warm fluid, some seven months in the womb. It's cosy and comfortable. There is an awareness of physical life. 'My heart is beating, I can move my arms and legs and turn.' Everything should be OK but there is also a background awareness of discomfort ... and an anxiety. 'It's coming from my mother and I'm not comfortable with it. It disturbs the serenity, the order of things. She's worried and I'm not really sure why. But it is enough to create an anxiety in me ... there are problems out there… there is now some uncertainty, something is not quite right.'

The birth experience: 'Head first and this is not at all OK. My head is sore, incredibly painful, mostly over my right eye. It is a piercing pain and it scares me. It seems that my head is being squeezed into a hole that is too small for it. There is also pressure on my neck ... and my shoulders. They're tensing up and it's uncomfortable. My head is turning now, and the pressure is mostly over my left eye, almost as if it's behind the eye. I'm moving but I have no control. I need it to stop ... but I can't make it stop. I need some breathing space - there's a sudden compulsion to breathe. But I can't. My chest is closed in, rigid. I notice my heartbeat and it's very rapid. I'm scared. In fact, I'm terrified ... it feels like I'm not going to make it ... whatever 'it' is. Alone. I peak with fear and now I'm angry. I am furious at this injustice, this restriction, my own helplessness. I can't move my arms - they're clamped against my sides. But I kick. It doesn't help ... anger fades, panic returns ... and a tiredness. I am really tired, exhausted. It's too tight. I'm too big. I can't get through. It seems easier, even essential, to just go to sleep. Forget. My heart beat is slow now, every time the squeezing comes. Ages pass. Then the pressure is easing from my head ... moving more easily ... an awareness of light ... hope ... fear ... and I'm **out**. I take a breath and try to scream my fear and anger. Gulping air ... my nose is blocked ... difficult to breathe ... it's **cold** ... people there ... someone - I don't know who - holding me. I feel alone ... where is my mother ... need her ... must have her ... confused ... she is life itself ... lonely and cold ... not good.

There is a problem with her ... she is in trouble ... she's sick ... I was too big ... fear ... my fault ... I can't tell her ... no love ... whimpering now ... afraid ... no hope ... there is a quietness within now ...

With my mother at last ... she's weak ... but it's warm ... it feels safer ... there is love ... feeding from her breast ... not enough ... still hungry ... crying. No-one understands my hunger ... sucking my thumb ... some comfort from that ... sleep.'

I was an eight pound baby and my mother had had a major post-partum haemorrhage. It was some hours before the bonding took place. I sucked my thumb until I was eleven years old and substituted that by smoking! But it wasn't only because of hunger - it was air hunger. From a big baby, I slimmed down and never seemed to gain weight. Even at fifty years of age, the suit I wore at eighteen still fitted me. It was as if I needed to remain slim for some reason. Now I know it was because if I had been any heavier or bigger as a baby, I might not have made it through at all. Cold feet and hands bothered me for years.

My guilt and responsibility problem had its ISE with the complications my mother experienced delivering me. It's easy to say today it wasn't my fault, but there is no logic at birth, only survival ... and I felt I might have compromised her chances of survival and her love for me. I needed that love to survive, or so I thought.

I had another experience of fear and separation when I was about eighteen months old. I was coughing and very hot, and had difficulty in breathing. I found myself in a tent with cold air blowing on me. I felt trapped in this oxygen tent. There was an overwhelming compulsion to get out but I couldn't. And I was alone. Very alone ... and terrified ... and 'they' were doing this to me ... why? ... a punishment? ... was I bad? That 'giving up' feeling returned - the Walking Zombie Syndrome, the acceptance of death.

I have been told that I had bilateral pneumonia, that the sulphonamide drugs weren't working, and that I was critically ill in an oxygen tent. They changed my medication to penicillin which was precious and difficult to get. I have also been told that I started getting better only when our general practitioner advised my mother to 'live in' at the hospital in a bed next to me. God bless that GP's insight!

This episode was another factor in my smoking habit in later years. It wasn't so much the nicotine, but the act of BREATHING in air and smoke that reassured my subconscious mind that I was alive and that I could relax.

Where I grew up we had some rough neighbours. Acceptance was gained only by daring feats and was always under review. At home, the family struggled financially. My father often was angry and I can understand his anxieties today ... but as a child, it wasn't at all easy to. I felt myself to be a burden, an obstacle - particularly with regard to the financial status of the family. This guilt led to my reticence in receiving anything from others - material things or love. I no longer wanted to be under any obligations because they threatened my mind survival. My brother was four years older than I and I had to keep up with the expectations of his group of friends - there was really no-one of my age around. My younger brother was no problem to me ... I had no sense of a loss of love with his arrival.

One way I could prove myself was through achievement - that brought recognition. I didn't have to try very hard either. However, achievement had its drawbacks. We moved to another suburb when I was ten and of course I attended a new school. Those first two days at the new school were like being an alien on a strange planet. I didn't know a soul, or even where the ablution-block was, and was too embarrassed to go there, anyway. It was a devastating experience of separation and feeling lost. Worse, I was placed in the 'B' class. Having left the last school at the top of the class, it was not a very positive move for a boy already feeling threatened. There were some really rough looking boys twice my size - the environment didn't lend itself to comfort. One of those 'rough' boys, though, remains a good and true friend today, and I have had the pleasure of returning friendship to him when he needed it.

It was soon apparent that scholastically I did not belong in that class, so I was transferred to the 'A' class after two weeks, where again I was subject to a new set of circumstances, protocols and people. At the end of the first term I came out top of the class. Oh Oh. Immediate rejection by the top five. I had outdone them. Flash back to my brother's friends disapproving of this clever young upstart. To me it was crazy that they should be so upset. I was just me, and I had needed to establish my worth, express my capabilities. But their rejection was hurtful. I determined at a subconscious level not to 'clean up' again and never made higher than third in the future. I had a problem with two teachers who disapproved of this upstart who often knew more than they. I learned to shut up and do the 'right thing', for survival. This series of events represented my SPE. I became an avoider of disapproval, not so much as an approval seeker.

The same year however, my class-mates honoured me by voting me as their representative to the annual Children's Day gathering of many schools - at which each class would present the monies collected for those less fortunate than ourselves. Before we were bussed off to the Great Event, we were examined by some teachers to make sure we all wore the correct school uniform - the school's reputation was on view, after all. One teacher looked at my socks in horror because one of them was a little rough around the top - some of the knitting had become undone. She announced volubly to the world in general: "He can't go like that! He can't get up on the stage like that!" To use a clichè -I fervently prayed for a hole in the earth to open up and swallow me. I was **shamed,** mortified. I mean that literally - I died at self-esteem level. The hole in my soul became a bottomless pit. It may not seem much to an adult, but to a child it was devastating.

I wasn't 'the goodie two-shoes' I appeared, though - I got up to enough pranks, as youngsters often do. I held my own, on and off the sports field and received provincial colours for sport. I was popular, what in the States would be called an 'all-American boy'. I **had** to be so. I sailed through high school and my compulsory military service, gaining a commission in the armoured corps, and was the leading candidate officer on my course. I was even offered a permanent commission in the army. Everything I touched seemed to turn to gold.

Until my second year in university. There was a great deal of work to get through, and I did fine. In fact, as biochemistry really interested me, I even came top of a class of about 130 students in that subject. Then one fine day, I was told to report to the professor of pathology. This was confusing and worrying, as I had been doing as well as most - I couldn't understand why I had been called. Nobody else had been. I soon found out why. He dressed me down in the most ungracious manner, ranting on about how I was wasting my father's money, that I should be getting better marks etc, etc. I stood there in a state of shock ... spiritually dead, because there was no justification for this tirade, this personal attack. I couldn't think, I couldn't move. Here I was, a really better than average student, and being blasted from a dizzy height. This rejection was a shaming experience that reflected right back to one of those teachers in primary school and I was shattered. It reflected back to the responsibility and guilt I had experienced after birth.

When I could begin to think some weeks later, I realised that maybe some concern had been voiced by my family. I had a strict rule of never working on weekends - I partied. I know now that they wished only for me to be a success. This perception - faulty or not, crashed down on me, like the walls of the birth canal. And I got as angry as I had been then. That was it. I became very depressed because I could not express that anger. I **was** a drain on limited family finances - which was one of the reasons I got married in my final year of study - my first wife supported us. From then on, I did the minimum amount of work necessary to pass. And it stayed that way in terms of studying until I became a houseman, or intern, when my responsibilities to my patients, my work and the ethic of medicine became paramount. It is ironic to me that holding such high ideals, I was to become a pariah of the profession.

The reason for my success in practice was not only because I was a reasonably good doctor ... I simply could not afford to have anybody think ill of me: I was a 'disapproval avoider'. If I got a call at 2 am to see someone who'd had a sore toe for the past three weeks with gout, I would go. Oh, what a wonderful doctor. I guess so. But at far too great a cost. I was too popular and couldn't say no. Eventually I had to do something to control my practice, so I increased my fees by about fifty percent. This was unheard of. Colleagues told me I'd ruin my practice, but it got bigger still. This was the situation then - an extremely demanding practice, a home situation which was unstable and the final crunch of the SIE. Somewhere, a crack opened. I could not face the ignominy of a divorce, wasn't even sure I could handle the separation. Immobilised into a walking zombie state, spiritually and metaphorically stuck in the birth canal, I gave up to the peaceful sleep of narcotics. The psychic pain was removed.

Some three years later I was 'rehabilitated' and reinstated by the honourable medical council and licensed to go back into family practice. I became involved in clinical hypnosis through the persistent nagging and persuasion of a friend. I had seen some pretty startling things he'd done for some of my patients. One of Dr Jules Leeb's patients was also a patient of mine - she required a hysterectomy and she insisted I be there to assist. On my arrival in theatre, there she was in what I presumed was the drugged stupor of the premedication. As I reached for her shoulder to reassure her I was there, Jules told me to leave her be, that she was in trance. I couldn't believe it because she was usually very anxious about surgery at the best of times. I checked her charts: no premedication apart from atropine. Wow! So, risking ridicule from other colleagues, I attended a basic course in hypnosis.

From that time, I have never doubted its potential and validity. I must say, in all honesty, that family practice was becoming somewhat routine. Modern medical practice in urban areas has restricted the scope of GPs. I used to do most of the confinements in my practice, treat all the pneumonias and so on. In the last five years as a GP, I did not do more than ten 'pap' smears. Previously I used to do that in a week! Specialisation has taken over. The child has an earache? Take him to the paediatrician, or ENT surgeon - why bother with the GP. Super-specialisation has come to the fore. Also, as a GP in a city today, it is difficult to find a clinic that will allow one to admit and treat one's own patient. So one may make a good diagnosis, then have to refer the patient. One gets a bit 'browned off' seeing sore throats and high blood pressure all day long. There is little challenge, little satisfaction. Also, to keep up with technological advances is a very expensive exercise - not many GPs have a treadmill or spirogram in their rooms: the cost far outweighs the turnover, if one is to practise ethical medicine. This is not sour grapes - it's an acceptance that the world changes. Sometimes that change is not for the best, but change it does.

A change for me was due. It was a powerful change. One which some colleagues did not approve of - nothing personal, just that it was 'unscientific'. Oh well, I guess it threatened some of them. They were just surviving the threat they perceive. It's OK. However, I am interested primarily in getting patients **well**, and this has provided me with more fulfilment than I could ever have imagined possible.

CHAPTER NINE

Case Histories : Asthma

Let us now examine some case histories. I have selected them from a broad spectrum of presenting symptoms and diseases, to gain a better perspective of these ideas and to demonstrate some areas in which they may be useful.

Asthma

Having looked at migraine already, let us continue with asthma. Asthma, as many readers will know, is a debilitating illness which has crises and quiet periods, but at best is always there under the surface, waiting. It is potentially a life-threatening problem, but with proper care the vast majority of patients can be quite well and participate in all activities of life. To achieve this requires education, acceptance and ongoing care: it needs motivation from both doctor and patient ... and it needs compliance, especially from the patient, with medication - both oral and inhaled. It most commonly has an inherited genetic background as one of the 'atopic' diseases, which include eczema and hay fever.

Asthma is characterised by shortness of breath, wheezing and coughing. These symptoms are usually triggered by a bout of flu or a head cold, with exercise, exposure to allergens - both atmospheric and ingested, and stress. The pathology in the lungs is the swelling of the mucous membrane lining the air passages, production of excess mucous and spasm of the smooth muscle around the air passages. This all results in a narrowing of the airway, with difficulty getting air **in** and **out** and is characterised by the wheezing.

Treatment is directed primarily at the inflammation which is causing the changes in the mucous membranes. Usually this entails the use of an inhaler to bring the medication directly to the area. This medication can be cortisone or some other non-steroidal medication, which will modify the allergic process. There are white blood cells, called mast cells, which contain tiny granules. When a trigger factor is present, these granules release their contents: the chemicals which cause the irritation. The anti-inflammatory medication reduces the likelihood of their release, as well as their effect on the tissues - the swelling and excess mucous production then decreases, allowing a wider, more open airway.

The second direction of treatment is to reduce the spasm of the smooth muscle around each airway so that similarly, the passage is opened and air can flow more freely in and out. This medication is usually provided via an inhaler - again because it gets to where it is needed very rapidly, but also because smaller doses can then be given. Of course, both types of medication may be given orally or intravenously in emergencies. The third direction of treatment is to identify the trigger factors for an individual patient so that they can be avoided, or to take steps to desensitise the patient with a course of injections.

The fourth direction is one which is rarely approached and not utilised ... until recently. This of course is to look at the patient's psychoneuroimmunological mechanisms - the bodymind connections - and deal with them. It is becoming increasingly evident that we shall have to do this more and more in the future: on the eastern seaboard of Australia and in parts of New Zealand, the incidence of asthma is close to fifty percent of the child population! In the United States of America some six billion dollars are spent annually on asthma management - and 'only' one billion of this is on medication! The rest is spent on hospital admissions, investigations, doctors and physiotherapy etc.

The incidence of asthma has increased with industrialisation and urbanisation, resulting in not only higher levels of pollutants, but also increased stress levels: we are exposed to many more factors which may trigger stress responses.

A study of 777 babies born prematurely was done by Dr A Lucas and his colleagues in 1990 and reported in the journal *Archives of Diseases of Children*. They were looking for factors associated with asthma. To their surprise, 44% of these babies, **who were born vaginally,** had signs of asthma. This comes as no surprise to the hynotherapist. I believe the vaginal birth experience is the classic determinant.

Our patient : Janet

Janet was 32 years old and had been in a relationship for less than a year. She felt estranged in this relationship, as her boyfriend had begun treating her like a servant who worked for him in the home soon after they moved in together. She had spoken to him about this but had been rebuffed angrily each time. She felt trapped, was nervous and very depressed. Her self-esteem was low by her own admission and she could not bring herself to think of leaving him, as she felt this would be shameful and that she would be seen as a failure. Her asthma required more intensive therapy as it had deteriorated simultaneously. Initially, she was also treated with an anti-depressant, to which there was a moderate response. As she certainly had reactive factors in her life at the time, she was also referred to a psychologist. She was not able to make a proper assessment of her own needs nor to act on them.

Her early history revealed asthma from the age of seven. She had had a tonsillectomy at the age of four and remembered that it was a gas anaesthetic delivered by a mask. She recalled being very frightened by this. She knew nothing of her own birth and while her parents were strict, she said she'd had a good childhood. I've learned that many people who say this are either loathe to say anything against their parents or have simply accepted their childhood as 'normal'. The question one must ask is: normal as compared to what?! Interestingly, when asked for her full names, she had omitted her surname ... an indication of an identity problem.

After six months of helping her maintain a *status quo* – 'coping' - with medication and traditional psychotherapy from a psychologist, a situation which really just perpetuated her pain, she was offered medical hypnoanalysis which she eagerly accepted, primarily for her emotional problems.

The ISE - Prenatal and Birth Experience

At five months *in utero* she reported feeling anxious.

T	: Are you picking up on anything from your mother?
Janet	: Yes. I'm not sure she wants me. She's angry.
T	: Who with?
Janet	: Someone else. It's not me. Maybe my father. They're arguing.
T	: Are you feeling any love?
Janet	: No.
T	: How do you feel?
Janet	: Worried. Alone.
T	: If you weren't there, how would your mother feel?
Janet	: Better. I'm a burden.
T	: How does that make you feel?
Janet	: Bad.

The Birth Experience

T	: What part of you is going first?
Janet	: My head.
T	: How does it feel, how do you feel?
Janet	: Sore. I'm scared.
T	: What is it you're scared of?
Janet	: I don't know.
T	: What is happening now?
Janet	: I'm stuck! Can't move!
T	: How are you feeling?

Janet	: Scared. Very scared!
T	: For what reason?
Janet	: I can't breathe! I'll die!
T	: How is your chest?
Janet	: Squashed. I must breathe!
T	: Can you?
Janet	: No.
T	: What's going to happen?
Janet	: I'm going to die. Tired.

She was, of course, subsequently born and able to realise in regression that she did indeed make it, that she was alive. However, she was physically separated from her mother which, on top of the fear of the birth experience - the DES - she felt to be acutely threatening.

T	: Any love?
Janet	: No.
T	: How do you feel?
Janet	: Scared.
T	: If she is not there, what will become of you?
Janet	: I don't know …
T	: Can you make it without her?
Janet	: I don't think so, no.
T	: What do you do?
Janet	: I'm crying. They don't seem to care. They don't understand.
T	: Go on.
Janet	: I'm quiet now. Sleeping.
T	: For what reason?
Janet	: It doesn't matter anymore. It's better this way.

Janet had had a threat to her survival once at physical level, twice at spiritual level with the **perceived** absence of love. The truth is her mother **did** love her, as she was soon to discover with the bonding.

However, the die had been cast. (This latter idiom I use deliberately, to indicate how literal we are without realising it!) However she had learned a behaviour of withdrawal from interpersonal relationships - to go to sleep.

The SPE of her Asthma - aged 4 years : the Tonsillectomy

T	: Where are you now?
Janet	: They've come to take me.
T	: Who?
Janet	: A nurse and a man.
T	: How do you feel?
Janet	: Scared. Mommy's not coming with me. I'm scared.
T	: Where are they taking you?
Janet	: I don't know. Away.

This kind of separation experience is not a good one for a child - it recreates the birth separation and there is immediately apprehension, with the perception of an unknown danger. A lot of this is determined by the poor emotional preparation of the child for surgery. Children should be informed in a reasonable manner as to what they can expect. There are books available to help the parent and the surgeon achieve this. Children need to know about anaesthesia, and what they can expect to see and smell in the theatre. They must understand that the people are professionals, who are there to help them, and that the masks are simply to prevent the spread of germs. The attitude of the staff is vital - a nurse or doctor who is authoritarian and unsympathetic will guarantee a difficult child. There are many professionals who do a wonderful job. Sadly, there are also some who should not be there at all. And the use of a black mask is simply beyond me - it is the one colour that is universally associated with death, by adults and children.

Let us return to our patient, in the operating theatre:

T	: What's happening now?
Janet	: They put me on a table. It's narrow. There are lights ...and people with masks.
T	: How are you feeling now?
Janet	: I'm very scared. I don't know why I'm here. I want my mommy.
T	: What do they do now?
Janet	: They're putting something on my face! It's ugly!
T	: What colour is it?
Janet	: Black! (she said with fear)
T	: What do you think they're doing?
Janet	: I don't know. They won't let me breathe! I've got to breathe!
T	: What's going to happen?
Janet	: I can't breathe! I'm fighting them.
T	: Go on.
Janet	: Tired. It's going dark. I'm dizzy now.
T	: What is happening to you?
Janet	: I'm dying.
T	: And now?
Janet	: I think I must be dead ...

With the blackness of anaesthesia she had the faulty belief that she had in fact died as a result of difficulty in breathing - a belief that needed to be removed. This was her second subconscious acceptance of death in a situation where she felt she couldn't breathe. She **could**, of course, but it certainly didn't feel like it to her. In this situation, the child is actually in an hypnotic state because she is totally focussed on the dramatic and dangerous things going on. Even if the child has developed the power of logic, it is relegated to limbo as she struggles to survive. Her subconscious mind has perceived imminent death - nothing else is relevant.

The SIE of Asthma - aged 8 years.

In her history she had told me her asthma started at seven years of age: the subconscious mind was more accurate.

T	: Where are you?
Janet	: In the back garden, with mommy.
T	: What is happening?
Janet	: She's hanging the washing.
T	: What is she saying?
Janet	: She's cross with me. She's shouting.
T	: For what reason?
Janet	: I haven't done my homework.
T	: How do you react?
Janet	: I'm crying. I feel bad.
T	: Are you feeling any love from her?
Janet	: No.
T	: Go on. What happens?
Janet	: I can't breathe properly - something is wrong with my breathing.
T	: What does it feel like?
Janet	: Whistling sound. Wheezing.
T	: Go on. What does your mother say?
Janet	: She's holding me. She's worried.
T	: How does that make you feel?
Janet	: Better. She's loving me again.
T	: Let your subconscious tell me is there a reason for the wheezing then? Any purpose?
Janet	: Yes. I'm safer. I feel better if she loves me. If I wheeze, she doesn't shout.
T	: Anything else?
Janet	: No...
T	: Well, you're breathing hard. Feel the muscles working. What does that tell you?
Janet	: I'm alive! (said with pleasant surprise)

T	: So?
Janet	: Yes, it also tells me I'm OK.
T	: Now go back to the very first time you felt this breathing problem. That's right, just float on back to that first time. It's OK now. Where are you?
Janet	: Being born!

She was therefore able to use her reasoning mind in the present to understand the real cause and purpose of her asthma, and to relate it back to the previous two occasions where she felt threatened and had difficulty breathing - at her tonsillectomy and her birth experience. She was able to realise that as an adult, she no longer depended on her mother's love to survive and could hence let this symptom of asthma go. She was able to see that her mother 'not loving her' was a spiritual threat to her survival and that she had reacted with a physical symptom, one learned in the birth canal. Her mother did of course love her. However, like so many parents, that love was conditional. From that day – twenty four years ago - she has had no medication and no further episode of asthma. For all practical purposes, she is cured.

Understanding her need for love as a baby and child, she was also able to accept her own independent and unconditional self-love and worth. She knew that not having done her homework was not the end of the world - it was forgivable. Her mother was over- reacting, maybe in her child's best interests. In short, Janet grew up. She cured her Ponce de Leon syndrome.

Not all asthmatics have the same subconscious mechanism for their 'disease' and I am certainly not claiming that all asthmatics can be cured in this way. However, there usually are significant events involving either a physical or spiritual survival threat. The events may also be related to socio-economic survival and self-esteem problems. The point remains, if one person can experience healing, anyone can, if motivated enough.

I believe it was Dr Bernie Siegel who said that 'there is not one disease from which some person has not recovered, even at death's door'. The purely scientific reaction to the above case was: 'Ah, that's nonsense.' Well, this patient is living proof of a powerful subconscious need for survival resulting in a biochemical cascade leading to asthma. A need, which once resolved, became obsolete ... along with the asthma.

Medical science, which includes genetics of course, has firmly categorised asthma as a genetic disorder, at least in part. It is one of the 'atopic disorders' such as eczema and hay fever or allergic rhinitis. I am in complete agreement with this statement of genetic predisposition. However, we have to look a little further than this sweeping and exclusive fact, because I can no longer accept it as the whole truth.

We know that one in every five admissions to paediatric wards is wholly or partly due to an hereditary defect, according to the Genetic Services of South Africa. One in forty babies born suffers from a serious genetic defect. One in fourteen persons will suffer from a genetic or genetically related disorder at some stage in life. At least five percent of all live births involve a minor or major defect of genetic origin - still higher in Canada, where the figure is one in ten. These are disturbing statistics.

However, not every child of a 'genetically compromised' parent will develop that disorder. The reason provided is that the gene in question is not a 'dominant' gene, or that the remaining recessive genes have 'variable penetrance'. In other words, some genes' ability to express themselves is somehow altered, so they may or may not show up in the child as a defect ... yet as an adult, that person may still pass on the potential defect to his or her own children. Nowhere in the literature can I find convincing reasons for this 'variable penetrance'. Strange ... and very convenient for science.

We have examined a patient with asthma who was cured. We have also briefly touched on Dr Michael Meaney's work which demonstrated that genetic expression may be altered by early life experiences, which is to me at least one of the major factors involved!

This is very heartening, because previously a person with a genetic defect, such as atopy, was pigeon-holed with a hard and fast diagnosis and no hope of recovery, only containment or 'palliation'. Now there is the potential to reverse the genetic expression.

We can also conclude that one has to be careful about what is said to a person - be that a patient or a friend. In this type of focussed situation a person **is in trance.** He is focussing on an issue that is of paramount importance to him. What he is told may act as a post-hypnotic suggestion. He may completely accept and believe that 'this is now the situation, I have this incurable disease. Or, I have failed this test, therefore I am useless'. We - those working in this field - are beginning to realise how negative this can be to a person in the long term.

CHAPTER TEN

Systemic Lupus Erythematosus

The next case history is that of a woman in her early thirties suffering from systemic lupus erythematosus, which I will refer to as 'lupus'. This disease belongs to the group of disorders termed the connective tissue disorders or auto-immune disorders. When I was a student, they were called the collagen diseases and include rheumatoid arthritis, polyarteritis nodosa and scleroderma. They occur more commonly in women.

These illnesses are characterised by the body becoming sensitised to its own tissues - an allergic response, if you like, to its own cells with varying responses of inflammation in those tissues. The tissues most commonly affected are the skin, joints and certain organs, not the least of which are the kidneys. However, literally any organ may be involved. These diseases can be devastating and even fatal: patients may die from kidney failure, lung disease and so on. Should the kidneys be transplanted, the new organ or organs usually develop the same inflammation.

When the joints are affected the inflammation causes pain, swelling and stiffness: as the disease progresses the structure of the joints is destroyed, resulting in deformation. These unfortunate people become less and less able to function normally.

Lupus in particular has a predilection for the joints, skin and kidneys, and is usually accompanied by an ugly rash with big red, irregular blotches. Lupus is not an infectious disease. The cause of these disorders remains a mystery to science. The course of the disease may be variable, with spontaneous remissions and exacerbations, but no-one seems to know why, except that stress can certainly aggravate the process. Depression is a common comorbid feature which is interesting, because most patients do not seek adequate treatment for this.

Treatment for lupus consists of drugs which reduce the aggressive inflammatory process, including cortisone and some of the drugs used in the treatment of cancer. Prescribed judiciously, they provide a great deal of relief and can maintain a patient in a reasonably good functional state for much longer than could normally be expected. However, there is a price to pay in the form of side effects from these drugs. Many patients may have only a mild involvement and may not require treatment at all. Overall, though, it is a most unpleasant disease and the predicted life expectancy is reduced.

If the disease is of moderate or severe intensity, the costs involved in treating it are enormous. The patient is often on medication on a continuous basis and may suffer side effects from these drugs which in turn will need attention: stomach ulcers, low white cell counts etc. Regular investigations by means of blood tests, x-rays and urine analysis are ongoing, as it is important to recognise any deterioration: the sooner one intervenes with drugs, the better. Hospitalisation is expensive and some individuals may require frequent admission. Once organ involvement has occurred, the situation gets worse. The heart and lungs can be affected, but kidney failure is the most common feature. These patients require hospitalisation into specialised units for dialysis. Many need dialysis for the rest of their lives in a specialised unit or at home, if they can afford it.

In short, this disease and its cousins are amongst the most unpleasant of illnesses and the cost to the economy is enormous. So ... can medical hypnoanalysis do anything to assist? Most definitely. Each lupus patient I have treated, **each** one, has had a clear-cut subconscious cause. Two are for all practical purposes 'cured'; they have been off all drugs for years and are free of symptoms. The others have responded in varying degrees and one not at all. The academics remain sceptical: "That's not much to make sweeping statements with." I agree, but they are still not prepared to do a study with me or with any colleague of mine. I have long since resigned myself to the fact that Academia is not prepared to cooperate with formal controlled trials.

I believe that most serious disorders have a major psychological component as a causal factor. I have gone on record as proposing that these diseases should be considered as 'malignant psychosomatic diseases' and that they are treatable, potentially curable with medical hypnoanalysis.

Patient Rose

Rose was 32 years old when she came to see me, referred by her doctor which was especially encouraging to me: at last, someone was prepared to have an open mind and act in the interests of his patient!

Asked what the problem was, Rose replied : "I'm sitting with a skin problem - you can see for yourself", indicating a raised purplish red spot, one and a half centimetres in diameter, on her right cheek and a rash on her arms. She continued: "I don't know - I seem to have been unhappy all of my life. Nothing helps anymore. I have joint and muscle pains which started when I was eight or nine years old - they diagnosed me as childhood rheumatoid arthritis."

Asked what she would do if the problem could be cured she replied: "Live with myself." This was an indication of her guilt and Identity Problem, and was exactly what her subconscious was preventing. Furthermore, her statement confirmed that she was already 'dead.'

The rash and joint pains had begun in earnest four or five years previously. Asked whether there had been any related events around that time in her life, she tearfully said: "My baby son drowned."

Going further into her history, I learned that she had had a tonsillectomy at about six years of age and a near drowning around the same time. Another important part of the history I elicited was that prior to the onset of her joint pains in childhood, she had been sexually molested by her father, who was often drunk. In general she did not seem to have been a very welcome child - her parents were unloving or certainly displayed 'conditional' love.

Her first sentence in the history was 'sitting with a skin problem'. Sitting - not moving, stuck. The prenatal experience already made her a candidate for the ISE, as did the birth experience - her first survival threats. This was known since the subconscious had already told me that she'd been unhappy 'all my life' – that is quite literal.

The SPE was undoubtedly the molestation by her father, for this was the precursor to her 'childhood rheumatoid arthritis'. In retrospect, it was clearly the onset of her lupus, which had resolved after a stay in hospital and at home. She had experienced period pains from the start of menstruation - another piece of the puzzle confirming the self-punishment of guilt.

Finally, it seemed clear that the tragic event of her son's death was the SIE.

The Word Association
    My problem = life
    The colour of my problem = black = death
    The emotion of my rash = guilt
    It all began when = father

So, her **real** problem was death and it was related to guilt and her father.

The Death Expectancy Syndrome
    When the walls close in = darkness
    Darkness = death
    If I don't get out = I'll die
    Loneliness = fear

The Walking Zombie Syndrome
    I'm just like = my father
    My father = dead (her father had died some years before)
    [ie : **I'm** dead! So there it is.]
    I was near death when = father
    It felt like I died when = my baby died

The Jurisdictional Problem
    When I die I'm scared I'm going to = hell
    I feel responsible for = everything
    Guilt = church
    My greatest sin = my whole life
    My punishment = sick

Ponce de Leon Syndrome
    Responsibility = you have to take it all on yourself
    If only = I could be a child again [!! - none of these responsibilities]
    Please don't = leave me

The Identity Problem
    Who = am I
    Need = love
    My greatest need = to be loved

    My assessment was therefore the diagnoses of the JDP, the WZS and an IDP as the major contributing factors. I have confirmed that the SPE was related to her father: since she remembered this molestation it could not, by definition, be the ISE.

The Prenatal Event

    Prior to her mother's awareness of the pregnancy, all was well. When her mother did become aware that she was pregnant the problems began. Her perceptions of her mother's reaction were that she had mixed feelings. She was happy to be pregnant but also sad: the reason was soon to unfold. When father found out about the pregnancy, he was not at all happy.

T	: How long have you been there?
Rose	: Six months.
T	: What are you picking up from your mother?

Rose	: She's crying. He's also there. He's talking to her. He's aggressive. He's angry.
T	: How do you feel?
Rose	: Scared.
T	: Is there anything you can do?
Rose	: No. Just hide away.
T	: Let the time pass. Go to the next important time for you.
Rose	: OK. Seven months.
T	: What's happening?
Rose	: She's fighting with my father.
T	: How do you feel about this?
Rose	: Confused. Alone. Scared. Sad.
T	: Are you picking up on any love?
Rose	: No.
T	: What are you going to do?
Rose	: Hide away.
T	: Emotionally, do you feel alive?
Rose	: Yes.
T	: Spiritually?
Rose	: No.
T	: Do you feel any meaning?
Rose	: No.
T	: Any purpose?
Rose	: No. Just to get out.
T	: What do you think of yourself?
Rose	: I'm in the way. I feel bad being here.
T	: What emotion is that?
Rose	: Guilty.

And there it is. There was no mystery, merely guilt in the prenatal event. It's so 'simple' as to be ridiculous, a term one eminent academician used. However, it was not ridiculous to Rose's subconscious - she had real threatening problems, she had **pain** and her inner mind was crying out for help. Working together, we were able to provide that assistance and heal her pain.

Interestingly, many patients with a rash or acne say in trance that they are hiding away from the world. Rose was to do that later too but it began, as we predicted, in the womb. There, she could only form opinions of herself according to her environment - there was nobody to tell her that she was OK, it wasn't she who was the problem; or to tell her that no matter what her parents said or felt or did, she was a creation of the universal energy we call God. It certainly wasn't her mother who selected that egg out of millions or her father who selected that sperm out of many more millions. There was no-one to tell her that despite what was happening, she **was loveable**. Instead, she formed the faulty beliefs that she was not loveable, that she was in the way, that she was the guilty party by just being there, that she couldn't like herself and that she needed to hide away from this threat to her spiritual survival. Being unloved was to her a death-like situation: she had already accepted spiritual death before she was born.

Here we find a common theme of feeling unloved and unworthy. To deal with this she chose to hide away and dislike herself - and as I was to discover, when "I am not wanted or have no place here, then I may as well just leave."

The Birth Experience

With this uncertainty, the birth process began:

T	: How do you feel?
Rose	: Uncertain.
T	: Of?
Rose	: Going out. The outside.
T	: What part of you is going first?
Rose	: My head. It's sore. And my shoulders.
T	: Go on. How do you feel?

Rose	: Scared. I can't move my arms. I'm scared to move.
T	: For what reason?
Rose	: She's sore. It's my fault she's sore.
T	: How does that make you feel?
Rose	: Guilty. Maybe she won't like me.
T	: Go on.
Rose	: I'm stuck. I can't move. I want to breathe. Scared.
T	: What is happening to you?
Rose	: I'm dying.
T	: Do you have any hope?
Rose	: No.

Rose had now accepted her own physical death. She was encouraged to continue and was of course subsequently born. The fact that she was indeed alive was confirmed so that she could remove the faulty belief of physical death. The immediate postnatal period was then explored:

Rose	: I want to be with my mother.
T	: Where is she?
Rose	: She's in pain. She doesn't want me. They take me away. To another room.
T	: How do you feel there?
Rose	: It doesn't bother me now.
T	: Why not?
Rose	: It just doesn't matter. I don't care.
T	: Do you feel alive still?
Rose	: No.
T	: Does that serve any purpose?
Rose	: Yes. I don't feel my pain anymore.
T	: Go to the first time you're with her. How does that feel?
Rose	: She pretends to be happy. But she isn't.
T	: How does that make you feel?
Rose	: Dead.

T	: Anything you can do?
Rose	: No. Just sleep.

Her reaction of escaping real or imagined threats, of hiding by sleeping was therefore reinforced. She contacted her mother who confirmed her own feelings at her birth. Already primed by her awareness of an angry father while still in the womb, Rose's relationship with her father was now one of fear, anger and helplessness rather than of love and acceptance. Rose was already viewing the future as threatening and unsafe.

These two events represented her Initial Sensitising Event.

As a child is growing through the early critical years, unsure of her safety, she **needs** to know that the love and caring are there - or all is lost! Rose was not often given that reassurance. The love that was provided was conditional on her fulfilling her parents' expectations. She had further events which consolidated her ideas of fear and death, not just emotionally but also physically: most notably, her tonsillectomy and her near drowning. We shall look at the tonsillectomy:

Age 6 years: the tonsillectomy and the DES with subsequent WZS.

T	: Where are you?
Rose	: In the hospital.
T	: Who is with you?
Rose	: My mother.
T	: How do you feel?
Rose	: Scared. I don't know what is going to happen.

[This is how she began in the womb - with an unknown future]

T	: Go on. To when you're on your way to the theatre.
Rose	: On a trolley.
T	: Where is your mother?
Rose	: Stayed behind. More scared now.

T	: Go on.
Rose	: In the theatre. Panicky. They're putting me to sleep.
T	: How?
Rose	: With a needle.
T	: Tell me what happens as the injection works.
Rose	: Going to sleep. Getting dark.
T	: How do you feel about it?
Rose	: Scared. Helpless.
T	: What is that darkness?
Rose	: Death.

So she had another acceptance of death here, 'abandoned' by her mother and in no control of her destiny. A similar sequence occurred with her near-drowning in a swimming pool, where she felt she had no chance of getting out ie she was **stuck** in a situation with no control - remembered vividly by the subconscious mind as the birth experience. The Symptom Producing Event - age 8 years.

T	: Where are you, Rose?
Rose	: In mommy and daddy's bedroom.
T	: Go on, what is happening?
Rose	: He's touching me [agitated]
T	: Where?
Rose	: Down there. I'm scared.
T	: Yes, you're scared. What could happen?
Rose	: He mustn't do this! It's sore!
T	: For what reason mustn't he do this?
Rose	: It's wrong. Mommy said not to touch there.
T	: Where's mommy, Rose?
Rose	: Not here. Out.
T	: What do you do Rose?
Rose	: I tell him to stop. But he doesn't.
T	: Do you want to go away?

Rose	: Yes. I'm cross.
T	: For what reason don't you go?
Rose	: He'll get cross. I'm scared of him.
T	: I see. So he carries on?
Rose	: Yes.
T	: How do you feel about yourself?
Rose	: Bad.
T	: Who is doing this, Rose?
Rose	: He is.
T	: So who is the bad one, Rose? You or him?
Rose	: He is. But I let him.
T	: That's right. You **had** to let him. You were scared, isn't that so?
Rose	: Yes.
T	: If he gets very cross, what could happen?
Rose	: I'll get hurt.
T	: And then?
Rose	: Die.
T	: So you had no choice, did you?
Rose	: No.

Rose's reactions were those of her learned subconscious survival techniques - when her fear did not bring about her escape from the situation, she 'went to sleep', switched off in this trap, powerfully reminiscent of her experience in the womb and birth canal. Nor could she tell her mother:

T	: Are you going to tell mommy?
Rose	: **No!**
T	: Why not, Rose?
Rose	: Because she won't love me anymore.
T	: And if she doesn't love you anymore?
Rose	: I'll die.

T	: Where did you first have that thought, Rose?
Rose	: When I was in her tummy!
T	: What are you going to do about this?
Rose	: Hide.
T	: Let subconscious tell me, does this have anything to do with your period pains later?
Rose	: Yes.
T	: What purpose did the pain serve you?
Rose	: To punish myself for being bad.

Rose had again experienced the fear of the Death Expectancy Syndrome and a loss of love when she most needed it. She became a Walking Zombie. At the same time she was now subconsciously in a perpetual state of anxiety as to her survival and had the JDP powerfully imprinted. She was able to review this situation and confirm to herself that she was guiltless - indeed she was doing what she had to - **survive**.

Soon after this she developed her rheumatoid arthritis of childhood - this had three secondary gains for her subconscious - it was punishing, she was removed from the threatening situation by being hospitalised and, importantly, she gained caring and attention.

As a result of her Identity Problem, Rose felt guilty by merely existing - the Jurisdictional Problem. She had judged and punished herself. Her symptoms served to gain her sympathy and attention; what she really needed was **love** and unconditional acceptance. Rose learned the reasons for her depression: she felt she simply didn't want to be here. 'If no-one will love me, I'll just sleep, I won't be here. I'll find a way not to be here - the illness will make me dead.' The Walking Zombie Syndrome. Subconsciously, she was simply conforming her body to the idea that she had in her mind - that she was dead! That she had no place here. Biological suicide.

As a child, her symptoms resolved over a period of two years and ostensibly she was 'cured'.

However, with her IDP, WZS and JDP, she was now set up for the problem of her lupus.

The Symptom Intensifying Event - age 31 years

T	: Where are you?
Rose	: At work.
T	: What is happening, Rose?
Rose	: There's a phone call. From the maid.
T	: Go on.
Rose	: She says to come quickly. Something's terribly wrong. My baby. She's taken him out of the pool.
T	: How are you feeling?
Rose	: Awful. Very frightened.
T	: Go on, Rose. What do you do?
Rose	: I get in my car. I just rush out and go.
T	: What thoughts are you having on the way? What is the paramount thought in your mind?
Rose	: His safety.
T	: If he is not?
Rose	: I'll never forgive myself.
T	: What do you find? You're at home now.
Rose	: [Tears and wracking body movements] He's dead. He's drowned. He's gone, my little boy is gone. He's so cold and still ...

Rose experienced the worst fear of any parent, particularly a mother. She felt a degree of guilt that to her was nightmarish. Though a logical clinical assessment obviously removed her from all blame, she was overwhelmed by guilt based on her past feelings of responsibility and self-recrimination. She died inside. She felt she no longer had any purpose to her life, and that she was indeed being punished by God for her past. She was a prisoner of her earliest perceptions.

Having accepted this internal, spiritual death, she proceeded to conform her body to the belief she held in her mind - and within weeks the symptoms of her lupus began. She had shooting pains in her face and limbs. Examination and investigation by her doctor revealed nothing in the early months. Her rash appeared, her joint pains became worse and eventually the diagnosis was obvious - and confirmed on serological tests.

Utilising techniques in hypnosis, she was able to speak to her little boy, to make peace with him, to find a closure. She was able to see how the whole tragedy of her own illness had developed, where the roots of guilt and deadness really were. She was able to understand with her adult rational mind that God was not punishing her. She had taken every precaution to prevent tragedy. It was **not** her fault. **She** was not dead. Of utmost importance, with this knowledge and recognition of her own good self, she was able to forgive herself.

A dramatic resolution of her symptoms occurred ... within the space of one week. With her mind-body connection in a positive flow, she healed herself, with minimal additional help from me.

She has remained well ever since, physically and spiritually. She radiates love - her love battery is fully charged and her subsequent children are reaping the benefits too.

Rose was courageously able to go back and examine some of the real reasons for her lupus. She was able, with great satisfaction, to say to herself: **"I love me!"** and recognise that she is a perfectly normal worthwhile human being. She was able to relegate to the past all the old faulty ideas – for example that her very existence depended on the whims of other people - and expunge her unnecessary guilt feelings. She was able to make the decision to **live**. To live with herself - remember what she said in the history? "If I was cured, I would be able to live with myself". She knew what her problem was all along – an amazing woman!

CHAPTER ELEVEN

Anorexia, Bulimia and Depression

Our patient this time is a woman whose problem of anorexia and bulimia manifested in her early twenties. Often, this is a disease complex which begins in the teenage years. All types of eating disorders, especially severe anorexia nervosa, have a significant mortality rate. The most common form of treatment today is a combination of anti-depressants and cognitive behaviour modification in an in-patient facility, with very close follow-up as an out-patient. It is a complex problem and a most frustrating and difficult condition to treat.

April came to me with the following story: "Well, I'm bulimic, but not as commonly understood. I binge and abuse drugs - any kind of sedative that will make me sleep and run away from the horror of bingeing. I used to be anorexic and then I felt fantastic. I'm told I've got a wrong body image by everybody - to me right now, I'm fat and I'm terribly distressed about it. I don't like to be told I'm looking well because that means I'm looking fat."

Asked for how long she'd been a worrier, she replied: "All my life". She said she did not eat at all when very depressed. "There are times when I binge and I don't know why - and that kills me. I've spent all my time drugged in bed, not able to work or run the house. I've been more in hospital than out of it. I've been pathetic. My life has been ruined - destroyed the last few years." She also had had migraines and was by her own admission abusing alcohol as well as sedatives.

I asked her what it would mean to her if she was to be cured and she replied: "I'd like to live - I haven't lived for ten years." It was evident that April had the Walking Zombie Syndrome, amongst other things. She was also a very angry person at times which is typical of the Ponce de

Leon Syndrome - she often provoked arguments, as she did as a child, especially if she felt her freedom was being threatened. Freedom was a very important concept to her: it was life itself.

As a child, her relationship with her parents was bad, particularly with her father who was "so loving" but at the same time very strict and a perfectionist. She felt that things went wrong when she was about ten or eleven years old and had treated them very badly. She became involved in a significant relationship in her late teens and early twenties, which had little future because of religious differences and ended some time after she had an abortion. The abortion was traumatic to her in many ways - in fact she said in the Word Association that it "left me so cold for so many years." She had felt no guilt since that time, which disturbed her - she could not understand why.

The Word Association confirmed the DES, the WZS and the JDP of guilt:

My real problem = me = sinner
My punishment = I suppose this self-abuse and destruction

The Initial Sensitising Event

She regressed spontaneously to six months *in utero* where she reported:

April	: I'm uncomfortable. I'm too big. My mother's uncomfortable and hot. I feel bad about it. But she won't let me out. I'm angry with her. I want to get out. It feels like the womb is closing me in.
T	: If you were any bigger?
April	: I'd suffocate. She'll have a miscarriage.
T	: And then?
April	: There'll be no more me.
T	: What does that mean?
April	: I'll die …

Small wonder, then, that she had an obsession about freedom and being too big ... the birth experience had the potential to intensify these thoughts, as well as her reaction of anger.

The Birth Experience

T	: What is happening?
April	: I'm protecting myself - I'm shrivelling up [!]. I'm being battered.
T	: How is your head?
April	: It feels squashed. It's too big. It's worrying because everything will be crushed. I'll be born brain-damaged.
T	: What are you doing about it?
April	: Push my way out - hammer with my head.
T	: Go on. What's happening?
April	: I'm impatient. Can't wait for air. Confined, restricted and stuffy.
T	: If you can't breathe?
April	: I'll die.
T	: If you were any bigger?
April	: I'd split her from end to end. She's very painful [sic].
T	: How do you feel about that?
April	: I'm more concerned. Coming out.

Once more, the usual manoeuvre to allow her to verify that she **was** alive was carried out. Then:

T	: What's going on now?
April	: They're laughing.
T	: And you?
April	: I'm screaming.
T	: Why?
April	: Because I want to eat!

T	: How do you feel away from her?
April	: Separated, estranged. I'm wild - I scream. Hungry. They wash me ... still screaming. Now I'm in my father's arms - nice smell.
T	: What are you picking up from him?
April	: Love!
T	: How do you feel now?
April	: Good. **I'm not hungry anymore.** (my emphasis)
T	: Go to when you're with your mother.
April	: Oh, it's very loving. Wonderful. But she's sad, so sad. I'm sad.
T	: For what reason is she sad?
April	: I have no idea. Maybe it's me. Bewildered.
T	: Anything you can do?
April	: Make her happy. Make her laugh. She's still so sad.

Now, in the history, we had established that her mother's own mother had died that day, or the day before: this was the reason for her mother's sadness, which increased April's sense of responsibility and need for approval and love. These events and her reaction to them became the basis of her pattern of reacting to future stressful events - or what she perceived as stressful events. A need for freedom extended to an obsession with personal space and control, and not simply a place as in claustrophobia. She felt that if her body had been any bigger, she would not have survived - and this formed the basis of her anorexia. If these needs were not met, she would react with anger, she would have to eat ... as she felt after being born, because once it can breathe the three things a baby needs are food, warmth and love. She would then sleep ... because this was what her subconscious perceived to be the way to survive at that time. These responses were not the result of adult, logical thought but rather of automatic subconscious responses. In such a situation, with the conscious realisation of her behaviour she would have to escape the embarrassment and her sense of failed responsibility - she would have to switch off somehow and this was achieved with sedatives or alcohol.

Symptom Producing Events

Age 4 years

Her first day of nursery school was a traumatic event which intensified her separation anxiety.

April : I'm frightened. The teacher looks like a witch. My mother and father have left me. I'm screaming for them to come fetch me. I'm alone – I want to be home. It's safe there. There's nothing I can do - no hope.

Age 4 years - the tonsillectomy.

T : How are you feeling?
April : Very strange. Alien. I'm clinging to my mother.
T : What emotions do you feel?
April : Fear!
T : Go to when they fetch you.
April : I'm screaming. Mother is left behind! I'm afraid. I'm alone.
T : Where are you now?
April : In the theatre. Don't know why I'm here.
T : Do you know anyone?
April : No, don't know them.
T : Go on. What is happening?
April : Mask. Over my nose. Smell - chloroform. Terrible ... going to die. Struggling ... to breathe ... fighting, kicking ... they're holding me down ... angry ... they get cross with me ... black ...
T : What is that blackness?
April : I don't exist ...

April had therefore accepted her own death after a great struggle to be in control herself and survive - a repeat of the birth experience which intensified fear, separation from the safety of love and her response of anger. Thereafter her behaviour deteriorated: she **had** to have attention.

Age 8 years

April	: We're in the car on the way to Durban. I'm trying to get attention - I was known as naughty. I'm asking for food from the picnic lunch. I'm not hungry because we just ate our breakfast - I want attention. My mother won't give me the food. [ie, mother won't give me love]
T	: Go on. What happens now?
April	: I nag her. Father threatens to put me out the car. I am screaming and crying. He stops the car and puts me out. They're driving off.
T	: How do you feel?
April	: Panic. Abandoned. I'm gone - they've left me!

[She had accepted her own death with those pertinent words 'I'm gone!']

T	: What's happened to the love?
April	: No love. No hope. They really don't want me. I run after them. He reverses. I get in. Chastened ... I'll have to be quiet.
T	: Go to the first time you felt this abandonment, this separation from love.
April	: In the delivery room. Crying. They think I'm healthy. They don't listen - I'm hungry! I'm angry! I scream!

April's behaviour pattern was therefore becoming not just 'child-like' but neonate-like: that is to say, her behaviour was that of a new-born baby! Her Ponce de Leon Syndrome was becoming fixed.

Age 10 years

April was masturbating in her bedroom when her father walked in.

T	: How do you feel?
April	: I jump up. Somehow, I'm feeling guilty ... or shame. I'm trying to hide. It's something that's only done in private.
T	: Does he say anything?
April	: Get up! I don't want to see you doing something like that again!
T	: How do you react?
April	: I feel like a naughty child ... caught out. Embarrassed. I don't know what I've done. They're disgusted.

April had again experienced rejection, a loss of love. Added to her previous losses, her parents' ignorance about masturbation created a crisis for her in terms of guilt and whether or not she was loveable. She didn't think so - she disliked herself.

As mentioned in a previous chapter, children masturbate from a very young age - it is a normal and natural phenomenon. Stanislov Grof reports that they may experience sexual gratification at birth, though this is not my experience. However, children most certainly can and do feel sexual pleasure, at least from the age of a toddler. How many fathers have been embarrassed by their daughters playing 'horsey-horsey' on their legs? The fact is, everyone in the room is embarrassed - they all **know** what the little girl is doing, but no-one says a word. They think 'Oh oh. Mr and Mrs X have a problem with their kid'. Nonsense. Parents must accept that this is normal behaviour and refrain from creating the conditions where both parent and child may be embarrassed in public. Sex education in terms of what is socially acceptable is required, in a way that does not make it negative for the child. Frank talk with a child can result in surprising co-operation, once they know they're 'OK'.

April's problems, however, escalated - her relationship with her parents deteriorated. She was in a conflict situation, needing to be independent and free, yet craving love just as powerfully. She was angry in many situations and then guilty for behaving so badly. She began to see herself as a failure in relationships, and believed that she would have trouble attracting attention and love. She felt more comfortable at a friend's home and spent a lot of time there. This led to her parents trusting her less and less and accusing her of being selfish, always wanting her own way, of being oversexed and so on. The more this occurred, the more she sought relationships outside the family. Her subconscious need was for love and freedom but her parents could not recognise this. While obviously concerned for her, they used manipulations and guilt to get her to 'toe **their** line'. However, her perceptions of abandonment lessened her trust in them - she had to find unconditional acceptance elsewhere: she was still reacting with the normal needs of a two or three-year old. Small wonder then that puberty was threatening to her - she couldn't grow up yet because her need for love was unfulfilled!

The Symptom Producing Event for her migraine was at 9 years of age. She was shopping with her mother in a department store.

April	: I don't like shopping. I'd rather be with my friends. I'm always against everything she does. [that word again – 'always': this was of course exactly how she had felt in the womb!] She's irritated. I'm sullen and angry.
T	: Go on. How do you deal with this?
April	: I feel as if I'm going blind. Panic. Heart is beating faster. I grab her. Oh! I vomit! [Migraine includes very often a disturbance of vision – an arc of colours like a kaleidoscope which spreads across the field of vision: so she thought she was going blind! Of course nausea is very common in migraine.]
T	: How does your mother react?
April	: She understands ... Oh, that makes me feel comfortable [!] She takes me to a little room. I vomit again. I'm frightened and ashamed. I feel bad.
T	: Go back to the very first time you had these feelings.
April	: Being born.

T	: That's right. Come back now, you're in that little room.
April	: Pain! From my neck to my head, on the left side, by my temple. It's throbbing, relentless.. It's the worst pain!
T	: Go back to that first time again.
April	: In the womb. Bashing my head to get out. I'll suffocate. I'll die! Dizzy. Nausea.

She was rapidly progressed through the birth experience again to realise life, to understand the relationship between the threat felt in the department store and that of the birth experience. With relief, she found her headache receding rapidly.

T	: What purpose did the headache serve?
April	: Oh, to **get out**. I needed to get out, away from my mother at the department store, to get away from shopping!
T	: That's right, and you don't need to do that anymore. You can just choose now to leave. You're not a 9-year old anymore. Was there any other purpose?
April	: Yes. To express my anger. And ... to punish me because of my behaviour.

April had now realised her Jurisdictional Problem - her self-judgement and own punishment which she decided she no longer needed. She realised the significance of needing to **get out** of that situation - that it was an emotional return to her need to get out of the birth canal, away from a threat.

At the age of fifteen, she began to experience premenstrual tension, and this represented the major Symptom Producing Event for the eating disorder:

T	: Is there a reason for these feelings?
April	: It's illogical. It's hormonal.
T	: Is there an emotional reason?
April	: Yes.

T   : Is it OK to let us know?
April   : I hate my body getting swollen! It's **fat.** I've got to wear a bigger bra. Oh... ghastly! Fat!!
T   : What will these result in for you?
April   : Failure. In every respect of my life.
T   : Which ones?
April   : Men! My sport. Acceptance ... it's very important to me. I'm not accepted by my father. He's always been scared of me having sex. He doesn't trust me. I'm angry with him. I lie to him. My life is a lie to him. It's [the premenstrual tension] punishing me for being ...
T   : For being ... ?
April   : For loving myself.

April had to be led to believe she not only could love herself, but **must** love herself. If not, she would continue to suffer, continue to seek that acceptance of her sexuality by her father – love, which her father could not unconditionally give to her. By growing up, she could not avoid getting bigger. To get bigger was threatening to her survival - she had to remain the child to have her need for love fulfilled, just as she had the awareness in the womb that to be big threatened her survival. The seed of the eating disorder had sprung up, it was growing and about to spread leaves while she remained a Ponce De Leon Syndrome.

When she fell pregnant, it was a disaster to her - a death-like situation. Marriage was out of the question - she felt it would be the end of her boy-friend's career, that her father would never accept him as he was not of her religion. She could not tell her parents - that was directly threatening to herself. She was getting **fat** ... getting **big!** She reacted with the Death Expectancy Syndrome of the birth experience and prenatal event – fear. Since fear did not aid her to escape the threats, she gave up. The Walking Zombie Syndrome - death acceptance, her life no longer worth living in this situation. She reacted with the Jurisdictional Problem - with such enormous guilt that subconsciously, she blocked this damaging emotion out completely.

Helpless, she had to allow events and other people to take control of the situation. A clandestine abortion was arranged and carried out. She was terrified, and did not in any way feel in control of the situation. A physical threat, a mind threat, an emotional threat and a spiritual threat were present. In effect, she 'died' but determined **never** to be out of control again. Clinical experience confirms this extreme need for control in these patients: controlling her eating was a proof of life. Lose control … well, die.

The First Symptom Intensifying Event

This created a conflict because, as a PDL, she was still missing the essential element of love: this event was the beginning of a separation from her boyfriend … something she experienced as another traumatic death-like situation. She compared herself to his other girl-friends. Her whole life, her value, her body, everything was determined by other people: how they looked, what they did. To feel just slightly heavier, bigger than one of them was … failure … spiritual and mind death. She had to stay thin, and small. She became anorexic, because she could not say, was taught never to say … I love me.

Now dead at spiritual and mind levels, she could only find proof of life at the physical and sexual levels. She stayed thin because that enhanced the possibilities of acceptance, and survival. At birth, her father's acceptance of her removed her hunger! In her quest for love and the security it would bring, she had several relationships. She could not feel guilt, because that was too threatening: she **had** to be doing this to feel alive! This behaviour was her proof of life. Without it, she was 'dead'. Indeed, when asked in trance how an affair allowed her to feel, she said: "Oh, good, **Alive!**"

The Second Symptom Intensifying Event

April did get married … and her husband provided the necessary acceptance in her life. However, she still could not tolerate being closed in, or controlled. If he took over a line of her conversation with others, she would immediately react with anger, for reasons we can now understand and, more importantly, that **she** can understand. The crisis arrived when they went on holiday with her husband's daughter from his first marriage. She represented a high-voltage threat - a rival for his love. April again reacted with anger, which she could not adequately express - she was in a Catch 22 situation. Trapped again. She needed and valued his love, but could not tolerate any competition, which was overwhelmingly threatening.

Her survival response had been learned in her earliest years. She withdrew. Feeling worthless and abandoned, she cut herself off from living - the WZS. She slept, she had no energy, no motivation, had no appetite. She **had** to be thin to compete with her step-daughter. Her anorexia surfaced. She became deeply and suicidally depressed. She could no longer work. She required long term medical, psychiatric and psychological treatment.

As her depression lifted, and she began to eat she of course gained some weight. Indeed, some of the anti-depressants of the time resulted in weight gain. This poses an interesting question. Was this a direct effect of the tricyclic anti-depressants, or, if they were removing the symptom, did the subconscious have to provide an alternative symptom? Either way, weight gain was unacceptable to one part of her subconscious. It represented a threat to her survival in the womb. A further conflict arose because at a later time - soon after birth - she had to eat to survive. A balance, a compromise had to be found: bulimia! She would eat junk food and chocolates and then vomit it all out. This endless emotionally traumatic cycle demanded some relief, as life seemed no longer worth living. Her old learned behaviour surfaced: to withdraw, to sleep - she began to take alcohol and sedatives in big doses. Her suicidal tendencies flashed from time to time as she attempted to conform her body to the picture she had of herself in her mind - dead.

She was helped to recognise the endless loop of hurt, anger and hopelessness. She was able to delete the faulty beliefs of herself and accept herself as the beautiful and caring person she is. A person who is normal and who was always normal, until her negative perceptions of events fixed in her mind and conditioned her to death-like feelings.

April arrived one day for her session to report that "For the first time in my life, I feel comfortable in my body." She hasn't changed that feeling, she **is** comfortable. Sure, she still had some hurdles to overcome - and her subconscious mind has graciously provided us, session after session, with more material to work through.

At the time of writing she had not seen the inside of a clinic for six months, whereas before she was more in hospital than out. She has taken no medication. She has been faithfully doing her hypnosis homework and applying healthy reactions to daily events or thoughts. She is more and more happy and contented. She has had far fewer troughs of depression and only one episode of bingeing, which she was able to terminate herself. She is alive and far more tranquil and serene, at peace with herself. She is more adult today than ninety percent of the people she meets.

Hers is a story of great determination and spirit. I thank her for the privilege of sharing her road to health and the accomplishment of her own personal triumph.

CHAPTER TWELVE

Depression

Depression is a common and debilitating disease, affecting not only the individual but also the family, and was probably the commonest disorder I saw in general practice. It frequently co-exists with many other illnesses - co-morbidity - and both psychological and physical examples have already been given in previous chapters. In terms of the cost to humanity, MIT and Analysis Group Inc investigated depression in the USA in 1993 - it costs that country almost $44 billion a year! Hundreds of millions of work days are lost. But above all, there is the deprivation of a decent, fulfilling life for some, or much of the time, to millions of people. Men, though they suffer depression as commonly as women, often deny that they have it, perhaps because they fear losing their jobs, or because it is an admission their self-esteem cannot tolerate. Sadly, this denial leads to much unhappiness in their families, sometimes to divorce and suicide.

It is not my intent to give a formal classification of depression, which can be found in the American Psychiatry Association's classification, the DSM-V. This is a diagnostic and statistical manual of psychiatric disorders which is used world-wide by the professions and is a useful tool to assist in the collation and understanding of our knowledge. It describes the symptom complexes that characterise the different problems, which are tabulated.

However, it does not assist the patient very much in understanding his particular problem, beyond the sometimes stabilising fact that he has a recognised disease and is not crazy. As often though, it may be negative for the patient to be classified as X or Y or Z. Norman Cousins describes in his book *Head First* that sometimes, when people are diagnosed with a disease, **more** symptoms flood in, because now they believe they are ill, and this is true of many people! Further, an approach that involves dealing primarily with the **symptoms** does not often effect a cure. By cure I mean a long term recovery from the symptoms. Medical hypnoanalysis recognises that emotional problems have a specific cause over and above any genetic predisposition - a cause which is subconsciously known - and deals more directly with the real cause. Dr Ritzman described this diagnostic and treatment dilemma well: psychiatric therapy is primarily medicinal. Psychological treatment such as behavioural therapy may also often help the patient deal with his symptoms, but does not cure the disease. The reasons are that these approaches fail to recognise that an emotional problem has a specific cause and are therefore unable to effect a specific cure.

In other words, one may see a specific diagnosis as a symptom only - the Real Problem is the cause. Depression itself involves many symptoms such as sadness, loneliness, tiredness, guilt, a sense of worthlessness. Sleep disturbance is a common presenting symptom, especially a tendency to awaken in the early hours - despite the overwhelming tiredness. Depression has been described by Engle and Schmale as the 'giving up, given up syndrome' and more recently it's also been called 'freezing'. Enthusiasm wanes, both sexual desire and performance may be reduced. Alcohol and drug use and abuse are common. Weight loss or weight gain may be a feature. Anxiety is often present, and usually precedes the depression itself, which is an interesting feature explained by medical hypnoanalysis.

In medical hypnoanalysis, there are usually at least three subconscious diagnoses: the Identity Problem, the Jurisdictional Problem and the Walking Zombie Syndrome. Dead people. They are 'dead' because they have accepted in their subconscious, during the course of a significant event in the past, that they have died at a physical level or have come to the conclusion that life is no longer worth living. They may feel life has no purpose or meaning as a result of a serious guilt problem from the past or that they do not deserve to continue living - which is a spiritual death, or spiritual WZS with a need to punish oneself. If anxiety or fear is a feature of the patient's depression, there is always present the Death

Expectancy Syndrome or the Separation Anxiety Syndrome, or both. Experience has shown that almost all of these people had a significant negative prenatal experience. Most of them are stuck at an earlier age emotionally and are thus Ponce De Leon Syndromes too.

An over-riding characteristic of a severely depressed person is the 'look' of death. Their expressions are bland, their faces and bodies are fairly immobile. They shuffle around. Sometimes their eyes are sunken and darkened with rings. They **look** pale and cadaverous. There is no sparkle in their eyes - it is quite apparent they have given up on life. They use words that describe the belief in their minds: "I'm dead tired, doctor...", "I don't care anymore." When asked what their problem prevents them from doing, they frequently answer "Living!" The clothes they wear indicate the mood of death – dark. They are often dressed completely in black. It's not the fashion of the day that dictates this colour because as they recover, and begin to feel alive again, they wear brighter and brighter clothes!

Without becoming too technical, and for the purpose of a clearer picture for the reader, I will describe three simplistic types of depression - a description that I found useful in general medical practice to explain depression to my patients.

One is manic-depressive psychosis or MDP: popularly called "bipolar disorder". Of recent years it has become the fashionable diagnosis and is classified into different categories – something I feel is just the dumping ground for many. Classical MDP patients go through phases lasting from weeks to months in which they are initially very hyperactive and lively - manic - thinking fast and often acting on impulse in a destructive manner, especially financially. They seem to have no insight into what they are doing. They will spend great sums of money for example, borrowing credit which they have no realistic hope of repaying. That is the crux – 'realism'. They lack insight into the consequences of their behaviour. They are unable to understand but are devoured by this need for **stimulation** and success, which in medical hypnoanalysis is their 'proof of life'. Psychosis generally indicates that a person is unable to function in the reality of the present. After some time in this phase, they will very rapidly change course by

180 degrees - sometimes overnight - and become extremely depressed and remorseful, even suicidal.

The second is 'reactive depression' and, as the name suggests, follows a specific event in life, such as losing a job, or a loved one. Perhaps even an argument may precipitate the depression. Very often, these people recover spontaneously within about six weeks and seldom require medication, but they certainly benefit from a listening ear and support. Their sleep disturbance, if any, may take the form of difficulty in going off to sleep. However, once asleep, they generally sleep through the night. If the depression does not resolve they are vulnerable to the next type and reactive depression may continue into a long and morbid illness.

Thirdly there is 'endogenous' or 'biochemical depression'. The word endogenous means 'from within' - no outside reactive factor may be recognised. Often, there is a family history of depression, suggesting a genetic factor. It is termed 'biochemical' because we know that it is accompanied by just such a disturbance - particularly with the neurotransmitters serotonin, nor-adrenalin, dopamine and others. What occurs, very simply, is that less of these chemicals are available at the nerve junctions or their transfer to the next neurone is compromised. The anti-depressant drugs we use either increase the production of these chemicals or reduce their reabsorption, so that more is available at the nerve junction. The results are good: we can expect about a third of these patients to recover really well, another third to some degree. A third of these patients do not do well with medication. The newer drugs have the advantage in that in most patients there is little or no sedation. The older drugs sometimes cause more problems than the disease, with people walking around in a zombie-like state.

However, I and others contend that we are treating the **result** of a problem - the symptom, not the problem itself. If you want a definition of depression, this is what I offer: *Depression is a failed Flight or Fight response!* When the subconscious is confronted by a perceived threat it initiates the flight or fight response – and if neither result in survival the last option is to shut down, withdraw … accept death, becoming Walking Zombies.

If we continue to deal with depression simply as a biochemical genetically predisposed illness it is no surprise that the recurrence rate will be fairly high because we're trying to manage the biochemistry and ignoring the subconscious dynamics which result in the altered biochemistry.

Results are better when the medication is combined with behavioural or cognitive therapy. In medical hypnoanalysis practices, one therefore tends to see those patients who do not respond to the above measures - the thirty per cent of patients who do not even respond to electro-convulsive (or shock) therapy. While I know that medical hypnoanalysis is successful in the majority of patients, it is common sense to use medication in the mild, moderate or severe cases of depression, purely from a cost point of view and most certainly in those who are suicidal and need urgent intervention. However, in those patients who require repeated hospitalisation despite adequate psychiatric therapy, those who require long term medication and those who require several drugs in combination, medical hypnoanalysis becomes a very attractive alternative: it is short term, usually successful, long-lasting and very cost-effective in this group. This doesn't do much for the manufacturers of those drugs, or for the hospitals ... but there it is: the patient certainly benefits! And that is the primary concern.

Patient Ken

I have deliberately chosen this particular case, because it demonstrates important peripheral issues - the involvement of the family and the dynamics of what may occur. It highlights the fact that in hypnotic regression we are dealing with the **perceptions** of the patient **and** the family - often not the reality of the situation. It will become clear how 'blame' and therefore guilt can so easily be thrown destructively around causing unnecessary pain for all in the unwitting games that follow. This case report is a tribute not only to the patient but also to his mother, who had the courage to look at herself and regenerate the love to allow her son to grow. This patient's story is one of hope, self-understanding and self-forgiveness.

The History

Our patient is Ken, who at the time of his treatment some years ago was 26 years old and a 'perpetual' student - not satisfied with one degree, he was busy with a second and unrelated course.

On being asked what his problem was he replied: "I'm very depressed and I don't sleep well - I sometimes have to sleep with the light on because I'm very nervous. I feel very **lonely** and I don't feel very good about myself. I **suffer** from anxiety a lot." I asked him how long he'd been a worrier and he replied "Most of my life. I'm very restless at home and I don't know if I need to **get out** now." He also told me that "every now and then **I go through** patches. I think about death a lot - it scares me actually." This had started after his brother's friend had been killed.

If we examine the words emphasised above, we see that '**lonely**' may indicate a Separation Anxiety. '**Suffer**' already alerts us to a guilt problem. He had a fear of the dark and used the terms '**get out**' and '**go through**'. We are almost certainly dealing with a nasty birth experience.

His relationship to family members had been strained. "My mom and I are not getting on well - she's overprotective. It's been **our whole life** and she says things about my girlfriend. I think she doesn't want to lose me. She is smothering and manipulative - she emotionally blackmails me with guilt. I'm confused about religion - I believe in God but mother thinks I'm a heathen. I feel guilty like some of the things 'you've got to love God'. That's rubbish, that God is a loving God. She tried to force me to go to a church group and I hated it but I'd go because she always made me feel guilty if I didn't. I am afraid of her tongue." His mother had discovered him masturbating when he was ten and smacked him. He had 'terrible headaches' and rarely masturbated because he felt guilty.

"I was very jealous of my brother - there was a lot of rivalry between us and it was me who usually got into trouble - she used to defend him against my father but not me. Once I said 'you hate me' and she reacted badly. She was **always** the one who did the shouting." Yet he also described his mother as loving and said that she often used to hug him.

About his own birth he reported that his mother had "had toxaemia and I was induced early. I was a forceps delivery." He had been breast-fed for a while "but she was starving me." His medical history included encephalitis at the age of eighteen months, a visit to a hospital at eight years, during which he was held down while he screamed, and a nasty reaction to a drug called metoclopramide.

This reaction is medically termed an 'oculogyric crisis' and is a most terrifying experience for the patient. The eyelids seem to 'do their own thing' and there is an involuntary turning up of the eyeballs in their sockets. Very often the patient experiences associated panic, believing that he is very seriously ill. This is very easy to treat, with rapid relief of symptoms once the diagnosis has been made. To the patient, however, it seems like the end is imminent.

He had also had an anaesthetic at the age of 18 and reported that when he regained consciousness he was terrified and kept asking if he was alive. The staff had laughed, not realising the serious impact the anaesthetic had had on him.

The Word Association Exercise

In terms of the Identity Problem -
    I'm afraid when = I'm alone
    Most of all I want = to be loved
    My greatest need = to be accepted
    My problem = me

The Death Expectancy Syndrome was strongly evident, especially with reference to the Birth Experience -
    When the walls close in = fear
    Down in that dark hole = fear
    If I don't get out = I'll die

My greatest fear = losing the people I love (which includes the IDP: to lose love was to him to die).

The Walking Zombie Syndrome
    I'm just like = nothing (spiritual WZS)
    Underneath it all = black … and …black = death
    ie, underneath it all is death.

The Jurisdictional Problem of Guilt
    My greatest sin = hurting my mother
    My punishment = feeling bad
    The greatest obstacle to my happiness = worrying about my mother

The WAE also provided us with the Symptom Producing Event -
    It all started when = my brother was born

Regressions

Before any regression took place, he came in to report he had had an argument with his mother, in which she had apparently made the following statements: "You're not reasonable or rational. You're on a self-destructive path. You're worse since seeing the doctor. You're a spoiled brat."

The apparent reason for the argument was that Ken had become engaged to be married the week before and felt upset that his family had not even given him a card of congratulations. I'm not sure exactly what he said to his mother, but whatever it was he said it without being aware that his mother and father had secretly planned a surprise celebratory dinner! Mother unfortunately reacted to Ken very negatively … a pattern which had repeated itself over many years. Games people play: if you 'attack' someone, that person will usually and instinctively become aggressive too – it's survival. Neither party understands his or her own reasons for this reaction - and certainly cannot understand the other person's reasons. Or if so, the inevitable guilt must be avoided. This is most easily and often done with anger.

Somewhere, the games - also known as 'song and dances' had to go, or both would succumb. We decided to continue, and he had his prenatal regression immediately:

The prenatal perceptions were wonderful, filled with love and mother's keen expectancy of her first child. However, at seven and a half months, problems began.

Ken	: She's scared.
T	: What of?
Ken	: Of pain.
T	: How do you feel?
Ken	: I'm not comfortable anymore. I'm also scared of pain.
T	: How do you feel about her?
Ken	: Responsible.
T	: If she has pain, what does that mean to you?
Ken	: Maybe she won't want me anymore.
T	:And then?
Ken	: Oh, no ... I'll die.
T	: Is there anything you can do?
Ken	: Stay here.
T	: Can you stay forever?
Ken	: No, but if I wasn't here she wouldn't have any pain.
T	: Do you have any hope?
Ken	: Yes. She loves me.

It was around this time that his mother began to have signs of toxaemia of pregnancy! One wonders where this originates – probably from the fetus, because soon after delivery, the toxaemia disappears. It is accepted today in obstetrics that the fetus is responsible for the toxaemia! I have had other patients in regression in a similar situation who have actually expressed the desire to 'not be' anymore. This is a direct result of the IDP and spiritual WZS. Tragically in this case, no disturbance was necessary - the origin was due to the perceptions of both mother and baby. Mother was experiencing (consciously or not) a threat to her own survival, and responded with fear. The baby was also threatened, with perceptions of physical death **and** the possibility of abandonment and spiritual death. To return to the regression, after some weeks had passed:

Ken	: She's sick. I'm sick. She's worried.
T	: What about?
Ken	: I might die! I feel alone.
T	: Go on. What are you thinking?
Ken	: She could die ... then I'll die.

Clearly, a conflict had now arisen -

T	: Is it safe to stay here now?
Ken	: I don't think so. But I don't want to go out. I'm warm here. But there's danger here.
T	: Anything you can do?
Ken	: No. I'm helpless.
T	: How much hope do you have now?
Ken	: None.
T	: What do you do? Give up?
Ken	: **No!** I don't know.
T	: How do you feel about yourself?
Ken	: Bad. Bad just being here.
T	: Do you feel any meaning for yourself?
Ken	: No ...
T	: Are you aware of any purpose?
Ken	: No.
T	: What colour would you give these feelings?
Ken	: Black ...

This situation was carefully reframed, allowing him to recognise that there was no malice on either side, that there was no blame to be apportioned to either party ... that it was an unfortunate set of circumstances. He now understood that for many months all had been fine, so it was not a genetic phenomenon: it was a **learned** phenomenon, and as such could be reversed. He was provided an opportunity for spiritual meaning and decided he could let go of the many faulty beliefs which had already arisen.

The Birth Experience

This followed the typical progress of going head first, experiencing compression of the vault with increasing fear. Because he was a nail-biter, I asked him about his hands as we commonly find these people could not feel their hands during the birth experience - the nerves supplying sensation to them are squashed and the blood supply is compromised. Not feeling their hands creates anxiety so when they are born, one of the first things they do is to bring their fingers to their mouths to make sure they still have hands! Hence the nail-biting in times of stress.

Ken	: My head's sore. It's getting squashed.
T	: Where are your arms?
Ken	: I can't move them.
T	: Your hands?
Ken	: Can't feel them. I'm worried they're gone.
T	: How's your chest?
Ken	: Tight.
T	: Are you moving still?
Ken	: No.
T	: And what do you think will happen?
Ken	: I'll die!
T	: Go on.
Ken	: No, can't breathe. Angry! Want to go back!

T	: Can you?
Ken	: No! Helpless ... I'm tired ... dizzy ...
T	: What's happening now?
Ken	: I'm going to die ...
T	: Any hope?
Ken	: No.

He duly emerged and was born and he was encouraged to realise that he **was** indeed alive and had his fingers intact. Then,

T	: Where are you?
Ken	: I'm alone. Cold.
T	: How do you feel about this?
Ken	: I'll die ... I'm **angry**.
T	: Where is your mother?
Ken	: She's sick.
T	: What's wrong with her?
Ken	: She's dying ...
T	: How do you feel about that?
Ken	: It's **my fault!**
T	: If she does die, what will become of you?
Ken	: I'll be alone ... I'll die.

These faulty beliefs were also realised with the help of the Word Association and removed. Then,

T	: Go to that first time you're with her.
Ken	: She loves me. I'm feeling love. Safe. But I'm **angry**.
T	: For what reason?
Ken	: She left me alone!

He was able to see that his anger, justified at the time by his beliefs, was really invalid, that his mother was entirely forgivable - she had not done this in malice. Also, at two months of age, breast feeding was stopped and this left Ken feeling confused.

Ken : I'm confused. I don't know why. Feeling bad, maybe it's me. Maybe she's sick again ... she's worried about me. There's not enough food. I could die.

The Symptom Producing Event - age 4 years

You will recall that the WAE indicated 'it all started when my brother was born'. He arrived for this session with the news that his "mother was speaking to me about my brother's problems. She wants me to do this, to do that. I don't do it, and I'm further away from him." He spent some time expressing anger towards his mother, and this was utilised in the session: he was regressed to any time of anger with his mother.

T : Where are you?
Ken : At home. I'm five years old.
T : What is happening?
Ken : I'm in his room. I lit the tissues.
T : For what reason?
Ken : I don't know. I'm angry.
T : Who are you angry with?
Ken : My mother.
T : For what reason?
Ken : Because my brother was born.
T : Go back to that time. Good. How do you feel about his arrival?
Ken : Excited. I hold him.

Ken now displayed facial and body movements of obvious discomfort.

T	: What's happening?
Ken	: She doesn't bother with me. She's not with me – she's busy with him all the time. She doesn't bother with me.
T	: How do you feel?
Ken	: I don't like him – he's made her change. It's his fault. I'm lonely. No-one cares.
T	: What do you do?
Ken	: They say I'm a big boy.
T	: Are you?
Ken	: I want to be a baby.

This was a most significant choice of survival. He needed love to survive and felt he could get that as a baby like his brother, as he had himself received as a baby. He was arrested in emotional development right there - the PDL Syndrome, forever seeking love from the outside. This explained why he was still at university - he had to stay at home!

T	: Will that help you?
Ken	: I want that love. No-one understands. I'm angry with him.
T	: Without the anger, what would you have?
Ken	: Nothing.

This is an indication of the use of anger in survival, as perceived by the subconscious. 'Nothing' is equivalent to emotional and spiritual death, to mind death, because he had no esteem of himself. Self-love and -esteem are encouraged by the manner in which our caretakers treat us. If their reactions to our needs are negative or are perceived to be negative, as a rule we begin to feel negative about ourselves, particularly if our behaviours result in verbal, emotional or physical punishments.

T	: Go back to five, you're in his room, you've set the tissues alight. Go on now. Who is there?
Ken	: She shouts at me. She smacks me.
T	: How do you feel?

Ken	: I cry. She says she's going to lock us in the house and burn it down.
T	: How do you respond?
Ken	: I'm sorry, I'm sorry.
T	: What are you scared of?
Ken	: We'll die. It's my fault. I feel guilty.
T	: What is it you need right now?
Ken	: Her to love me.
T	: Go back to the very first time you needed that.
Ken	: In the hospital. I'm alone. I'm hungry for my mother. For love.
T	: Where is she?
Ken	: She's sick.

Ken was able to realise that his brother's arrival was a survival threat to him, regenerating the fears and guilt **and** anger he had felt with the Separation Anxiety at birth. He was able to understand his action of lighting a fire, and realised that his mother's response, though drastic in the extreme, resulted in his not lighting fires again, a good thing! However, the use of guilt to manipulate Ken had very long-lasting effects: he now believed he would never regain his mother's love and became a spiritual WZS with the guilt of the JDP. His protection - his Proof of Life - was of course, anger. During this session he retained a great deal of anger which he was not yet prepared to express. He did this at home, apparently, with unfortunate results ... but this was probably necessary in the subsequent unfolding of events.

I received a phone call from his mother before his next appointment, in which she had this to say:

"I'm stopping Ken's treatment. I've told him he can't have the credit cards, or the car. I've stopped his allowance because of the hurtful things he says to me. He's angry and I won't have it - he says horrible things and I won't allow him to carry on. I've been a loving mother and I don't deserve this. He's getting worse, not better. He was such a loving, compliant child."

Well ... this outburst revealed a great deal. In the first place, mother was very angry and she was transferring this anger to me - known as negative transferrence - as mentioned in a previous chapter. It also describes the way in which most mothers of her generation would have reacted, a generation strongly influenced by Calivinist beliefs, whether Christian, Jewish or whatever. Western civilisation has many social characteristics which originated in the teachings of John Calvin and Martin Luther. Apart from the obvious religious influence of 'honour thy Mother and Father', parenting embraced the concepts of 'children should be seen and not heard', 'spare the rod and spoil the child' and so on. The work ethic, the basis of the success of capitalism - is owed to Calvin. However, so is the fact that parents became more and more removed from their children and each other in terms of displaying love. Hugs were a 'no-no': any show of affection was frowned upon as being not in keeping with being one of the 'Elect', though most people were not aware of this religious aspect. Children were seen as **possessions** - they 'should be seen and not heard'.

Small wonder that mother was angry. Her son was displaying anger which had been internalised since the prenatal period: he was asserting his **own** personality. However, this was contrary to her own upbringing - **her** parents would probably not have stood for this! She had been sent to her room as a child, after all. This by the way, is metaphorically like sending the child back into the birth canal, from which she can see no escape, where she is alone and without love, the very thing she needs! Unfortunately, mother's parents had thereby stifled her own personal growth ... her anger was that of her inner child ... and hence, mother was also a Ponce de Leon Syndrome, the product of a difficult and unloved childhood. It is not the adult part of a parent which reacts to her own in this fashion - decidedly not - her inner child was being **threatened!** And she said some unfortunate things to her son Ken ...the song and dance was on ... in a vicious circle in which there could be no winner.

This was tragic because each had a deep love for the other. They were trapped in their own **perceptions** of their respective early lives. Once this fact of acting on subconscious survival impulse was explained to mother, and that Ken was now venting necessary anger, and essentially

PRISONERS OF OUR PERCEPTIONS

no-one was at fault, mother became her adult self and understood the self-destruction in their relationship. **This took courage** ... a remarkable woman to have achieved this in an impersonal five minute telephone call. However, her courage was the turning point not only for Ken, but for the entire family, for in the next session, Ken was at last able to rid himself of all his previous anger. Utilising his anger and what is called an 'affect bridge' to take him back to its origin, he regressed back there.

Not surprisingly, his anger originated in the prenatal experience and lo and behold - he wasn't angry with his mother - he was angry with **himself!** After all, he had revealed the Word Association 'my problem = me'! So, mother had also been right when she had told Ken he was on a self-destructive path. When he realised his faulty belief that he was hateful, when he realised the miracle of his existence as a product of God, a most gratifying mini-miracle occurred. He said after the regression: "I feel as if a weight has been lifted - I want to go home and cry, but I feel much better."

After the next session, in which he was given information about relationships and how to respond to the world around him, he said "I don't think I need to see you anymore."

He was now aware of the impact of the emotional perceptions in the PNE and Birth Experience, as well as the reasons for his acceptance of death. His guilt, which had revolved around his mother, had been understood and eliminated. He was no longer angry with himself. Indeed, he was able to joyfully verbalise 'I love me'! The family grew closer, tensions dissipated. Love feeds on love ... it is what we are all about.

His depression disappeared almost overnight and is unlikely to return unless he experiences a really severe Symptom Intensifying Event in the future. Should this occur, I doubt that it would require more than one session to resolve.

CHAPTER THIRTEEN

Post-traumatic Stress Disorder

Post-traumatic Stress Disorder or PTSD is a particularly disturbing condition characterized by intense fear, which often profoundly changes a person's personality and life. PTSD follows, as the name suggests, a traumatic event which involves a death or the imminent possibility of death or serious physical harm. It may be actually experienced or simply witnessed by the patient, who as a rule is not in a position to intervene in the course of the traumatic event: he or she feels helpless.

The predominant symptom is that of intense anxiety or panic. A number of associated symptoms may also be present - about half of these unfortunate people suffer from significant depression. They have intrusive thoughts of the event, as if they are re-experiencing it, which may also occur in dreams. Of course, any of the physical symptoms associated with fear can affect them, such as palpitations, hyperventilation, etc.

They often begin avoidance behaviour - keeping away from anything that may trigger the memory of the event recurring. This avoidance extends to emotions, and they may use prescribed or illicit drugs or alcohol to avoid thinking of it. They may decrease their involvement in activities with the family or community. Many of these patients have a feeling that they have not much longer to live, their expectations of life are diminished and they seem to have lost the ability to provide or receive love and affection. They often display unusual anger, are 'jumpy' and have difficulty sleeping.

Clearly, others are severely affected as well - in particular the patient's family and co-workers. Not uncommonly relationship problems surface, divorce is more common and they are likely to have difficulties at work, to the extent of dismissal. Not a pretty picture - there is a significant change in their thinking, emotion and behaviour which is distressing to all.

Traditional treatment consists of early psychological intervention with behavioural and cognitive techniques, and assistance in problem-solving for the whole family. This is a costly multi-disciplinary approach and indeed traditional psychiatry and psychology have stated that there is no 'specific cure' – our experience rejects this idea. Yet, once more, these unfortunate people are labelled sometimes for life since their prognosis is considered to be poor.

In terms of medical hypnoanalysis though, the dynamics can be simplified for the patient to very easily understood levels, in which a cure can certainly be achieved. In fact, a return to normal is expected, and one is very disappointed if this does not happen.

What the patient has experienced in this traumatic event is a Symptom Intensifying Event of the Death Expectancy Syndrome and the Walking Zombie Syndrome, and not uncommonly the jurisdictional problem of Guilt.

Of course they will avoid any reminding triggers! The subconscious mind, unable to use logic except for 'is this life or is this death' and, unable to change the negative train of thought, will continue to act as if the threat is still active and protect the individual from exposure to the threat or from anything that it perceives as re-igniting the threat of dying. It is reacting with all the energy of the **original** event, as if the original event **is** the threat now, because it does not yet know it is of no consequence anymore. And it will go on providing the flight or fight response in an endless loop - it can do nothing else. There is present an instinctual subconscious **compulsion** to avoid danger.

However, if the patient can be assisted in recognising the real problem and can understand that what he is doing is reacting to a **memory**, he should be able to cure himself! Let us see ...

Case study - Max

Max was a big powerful young man in his early twenties. I have chosen his case because his Initial Sensitising Event was a little different from those we have already examined. It was certainly his birth, but he was delivered by an elective Caesarian section ie a planned non-emergency operation. The reason for this was that his mother had had a Caesarian section with her first child, and now was carrying twins. The risks of the operation were considered to be less than a trial of labour in a vaginal delivery.

The History

"Um, I would say, I'm worried about things. I'm more nervous. I'm **always** on edge and worried what I'll miss **by not going out**. (My emphasis, the reason for which will become evident)! I've had one or two flashbacks and now I check everything's OK."

The word 'always' was the clue to the Initial Sensitising Event and I was curious as to his statement about what "he'd miss by not going out." I had a gut feeling it had to do with the ISE. His behaviour had obviously changed and he was tending to become obsessive about his safety.

What had precipitated his Panic Disorder was that he had been held up at gun point in the restaurant where he worked, some five months before. This was clearly the Symptom Intensifying Event. He also said that he had headaches, shortness of breath, excessive sweating and one episode of dizziness. He had lost ten kilograms since the hold-up and also suffered from diarrhoea.

The history of the Caesarian birth was obtained, plus the fact that he was the second twin born, by some minutes. He had had an operation for a hernia at the age of four or five years and two near-drowning incidents - one at five years in a pool and another at about sixteen, when he had been dragged by a rope behind a yacht at sea.

The Word Association Exercise
> Suffocate = claustrophobia
> Down in that dark hole = petrified
> I've just got to = get out
> If I don't get out = I might never
> My greatest fear = to die
> Fear = scared
> Death = scared
> The colour of my problem = off-red
> The colour off-red means to me = death
> I was near death when = a man held a gun to my head

Well, that seemed impressive to me and pretty straight-forward. The problem, of course, was death! Nothing strange about that and we don't require some cascade of psychoneuroimmunological or genetic mechanism to understand it. It's logical.

It was indeed straight-forward, given the genuine desire to be better by both his conscious and subconscious minds!

The Prenatal Event

The prenatal experience was generally good - he experienced consistent and spontaneous love from his mother, and the fact that he was a twin was in no way threatening to him - rather the opposite. There was, however, some uncertainty because his mother became 'naturally' anxious about delivering twins. Max was aware that she was anxious for **him** and his brother! He was in turn feeling responsible for her emotions and was only mildly uncertain about himself. All this was present from the fifth through to the eighth month, when she was informed by her obstetrician that a Caesarian section would be done with an epidural anaesthetic. This allayed her anxiety for her twins and subsequently Max felt calmer too. His spiritual self and right to be was reinforced.

The Initial Sensitising Event

Max was asked to go to that time of his birth and consented.

Max : It's time to leave. It takes time.
T : What is happening?
Max : There's a lot of noise ... from the outside.
T : Go on.
Max : Feeling claustrophobic - I want to get out!
T : What is it you're scared of?
Max : If I don't get out I'll die!
T : What is happening in the womb?
Max : It's open. My heart is starting to race. My muscles are weak. I haven't moved around enough.
T : Where's your brother?
Max : He's already out. I'm uneasy.
T : For what reason? (I was curious - there were no contractions or other apparent dangers).
Max : I'm alone. Maybe they don't know I'm here! Claustrophobic! I don't think they're going to take me out! Breathing fast! **Now** they take me out!

Max had been under the impression they might not have known about him, and might have left him there for good - he felt trapped and utterly helpless, all alone. Once he realised Life and this had been imprinted, he was reminded of what he had said to me in the history - "I'm always worried about what I'll miss **by not going out!!**" And of course he now understood - he **knew,** and with that insight, he smiled. His experience demonstrates that babies born by Caesarian section do not necessarily escape the Birth Anoxia Syndrome or Death Expectancy Syndrome. The regression then continued:

Max : I'm alive! My dad's looking at us.
T : How do you feel being away from your mother?

Max	: Still safe. Happy. (Of course, now that he was out!) My mother wants to look.
T	: Are you warm? Cold? What?
Max	: A little cold - not so happy. They're letting my mother see us.
T	: And?
Max	: **Safe.** She's tired. **Love.**
T	: Yes. Go on now, what happens?
Max	: They take us away to a room. Insecure! Love is too far away. I think I'm going to be left there. She'll never come back! I'll lose my parents.
T	: Can you survive without them?
Max	: Can't make it without them.
T	: How is your brother? Are you aware of him?
Max	: He's happy.
T	: Go to that time she's with you.
Max	: Better. She's around us all the time. Great.

'Caesar' babies also have the Separation Anxiety Syndrome - and it was more intense for Max than it had apparently been for his brother - which seems logical because as Max had been 'left' in the uterus, he was more vulnerable to separation! Knowing all this was the foundation for Max to begin healing himself.

The Symptom Producing Events

There were two of these, early in life and we predicted them from the history.

Surgery at the age of four years.

Max is in the hospital:

Max	: It's a big cream room - lots of kids there. Mother is there.
T	: How are you feeling there?

Max	: Scared. I don't know why I'm there. My mother's got a colouring book for me. I put on this funny suit. I feel naked ... uncomfortable.
T	: Go on.
Max	: Nurse comes in. Going somewhere.
T	: Where is your mother?
Max	: Not here. Scared ... don't know what's going to happen.
T	: Go on.
Max	: On the table. This big black thing. Doctor giving ... I try my hardest to not ... no power over it ... colours, green red, blue ... I don't ...
T	: What's happened to you?
Max	: I don't know. It's dark.
SPE	: Near drowning, age five years.
Max	: My brother and sister. My mother. We're sitting with mother at the pool. We go to the water. I followed my sister into the deep water ... **claustrophobia!** ... I could drown...die ... trying to come up for air ... can't ... I think I'm going to drown ... helpless ... mother pulls me out ...

Max had endured two threats to his physical survival and in each one he was not in a position of control. The operation was not a real threat to his survival - there were professionals there for him. However, that was not his perception at all. Indeed, he tried to not breathe the gas from the mask - the 'big black thing'. As far as he was concerned, this was a direct and immediate threat to his survival. The near drowning allowed the same thoughts and emotions to maximise and imprint, because he was in a hypnotic trance at the time, being so focussed on the danger. As a result, during this event he had images imprinted in his mind of fear, of loneliness, of helplessness and of death.

The First Symptom Intensifying Event

Max is 16 years old and sailing with others on a yacht.

Max	: I tie a rope to my back because the wind is very strong. We come around the island ... strong gust of wind ... pulled down into the water ... I can't help myself ...
T	: What are you thinking?
Max	: I think I'm going to drown. There's death around ... nothing I can do ...
T	: What do you mean?
M	: I'm going to die ...

His uncle however pulled him in and once more we were able to help him delete this faulty belief of hopelessness, of death and replace it with the certain knowledge of his survival. He was able to finally leave this incident in the past and with this done we could now review his final SIE.

The Second Symptom Intensifying Event

Max is in the restaurant where he works.

Max	: I'm on the till. I turn around ... there's this big guy ...stands over me ... climbs over ...
T	: Go on.
Max	: A little guy too ... three others ... he holds a gun at my chest ...
T	: How do you feel?
Max	: Disbelief.
T	: Feel your body now, what's happening?
Max	: My heart is racing, I'm tense - my muscles, my breathing is more ...
T	: That's right. Your subconscious is working for you. Go on.

Max	: He tells me to take the money out. I open the till …little guy takes the money … they want to go to the safe … they know where they're going …
T	: How do you feel? Is there anything you can do?
Max	: No. No control at all. There's a gun and a knife on me. But it's like I'm calm.
T	: That's right. Your subconscious knows there is nothing you can do. Nothing you should do except listen to them. Your interest is to survive. That's all. It's your only duty right now. Go on now.
Max	: The door is locked. I scream to the manager to open the door slowly … there's a gun at my back **… I think he's going to shoot …**
T	: He doesn't. He doesn't shoot. Go on!
Max	: Lies me down … gun at my head … one pull of the trigger I'm dead for sure … takes money … have to reboot the computer … security guard might see them … they're agitated … he swings at me with a knife … on to ground … kicked … I'm **angry** … trying to think of escape …locked in the storeroom …

Max saw that at one point he had given up any hope of survival, he realised that his anger had helped provide the stimulus to continue. He was given the opportunity to express that anger - which he certainly could not do at the time without certain death. He was able to realise he had lived through this horrific experience, that the danger was no longer active. More importantly, he was able to relate his physical, mental and emotional reactions to his ISE - his birth, and the intervening SPEs … he connected them all and saw that his recent symptoms were 'merely' his subconscious mind trying to make sure he was alive … that it was no longer a valid exercise because he **is** alive.

He was asked to make a formal decision to live and with that his problem was over. All that remained was to reinforce what he had learned and his ability to now choose how to feel, how to think, how to be.

CHAPTER FOURTEEN

Panic Disorder

Panic Disorder can be most debilitating and is, of course, one of the many anxiety syndromes that occur. Incredibly, one of the articles I reviewed states that a patient "suffers an average of twelve years before they are finally given the correct diagnosis!"

Panic Disorder is recognised in a patient who has sudden and unexpected panic attacks, though these may be triggered by some event or circumstance. Very often they occur without any warning. The patient experiences a rapid rise in the intensity of panic and for the diagnosis to be accurate, must have at least four of the following symptoms which are mostly the result of adrenalin and noradrenaline being released in the flight or fight response. As we considered in our model of the hunter confronted with the sabre-tooth tiger, this is a survival response and is governed by automatic subconscious forces.

There may be shortness of breath with a feeling of suffocation - a choking sensation which you can by now recognise as the physical feelings encountered in the birth canal - usually our first physical survival threat. There may be palpitations - the heart beating more rapidly and usually more powerfully. Shakiness, sweating, nausea or abdominal discomfort, dizziness, numbness, hot flushes may all occur.

It is interesting to explore the dizziness and numbness, because these are commonly present in the birth experience, but in a panic attack the recreation of these symptoms has a different mechanism: in the birth canal, the baby's oxygen levels are reduced, whereas in a panic attack the levels are high. This is due to the 'hyperventilation' precipitated by the compulsion to get air. The subconscious mind is regenerating the precise conditions of the struggle in the birth canal because it presumes 'if I felt like that with my first threat, and I **did** survive, then that's how I must get through **this** threat.' The difference of course is that in the here and now, there is **no** threat. However the subconscious, not able to think logically, provides a sensation of choking, called globus hystericus, which compels the patient to breathe - to **over**breathe. He simply **must** have oxygen.

As the oxygen levels rise, the patient becomes not only dizzy, but gets numb and tingly fingers too. This creates more panic because he or she now thinks 'I'm having a stroke' or something like that. In a panic attack, sometimes the oesophagus or swallowing tube goes into spasm because of the overload of messages pouring down the automatic nervous system. This presents as chest pain not unlike a heart attack, but has nothing to do with the heart. However, that's the first thing that comes to our unfortunate patient's mind and his flight or fight response is continued.

There is of course a **fear** of **dying** - and this is the core of the problem: the Death Expectancy Syndrome. However, most of these patients also have an Identity Problem. The patient may also fear he is going crazy, because the physical things that are happening to him are beyond his control. He may even feel he is losing touch with reality or as if he is disembodied, detached from himself.

It is a serious disorder because not only does it affect his lifestyle, but other associated problems often co-exist, such as addiction, especially to alcohol, and phobic anxieties, particularly social phobia. Often significant depression occurs. From the point of view of medical hypnoanalysis, this is predictable ... if the patient continues to have all this anxiety and fear, and seems unable to **escape** the fear sooner or later a sense of hopelessness will ensue as he gives up ... and becomes a walking zombie! Particularly so if with an IDP, he has no foundation of security.

Since he cannot escape his perceived threat (there is nothing to escape from) he may well develop the idea that he is not going to get better, especially if he cannot function at work because of panic. He sees his whole world crumbling and there is nothing he can do! He may then accept his own 'death' in his mind. Tragically, this is the cause of the suicide risk in these patients. Essentially, suicide is a 'logical' conformation of the body to the idea the patient already has in his mind - since he believes himself to be dead, it would seem 'natural' for his body to be the same and escape this misery.

The traditional management of Panic Disorder is primarily with medication, preferably in conjunction with psychotherapy, especially behaviour modification and cognitive techniques. The results are good but not ideal and may carry problems. Some patients - about a third of the total - may safely be weaned from the medication and remain well. There are those who relapse quite dramatically as a 'rebound' phenomenon, which may be due in part to withdrawal symptoms as they come off their drugs and finally there is a group who may require life-long medication. This is not a happy state of affairs because many of them loathe being dependent on the drugs and the potential for escalation of the dose is present, especially if family, friends and even professionals tell them to "come on now, pull yourself together!" This group has a higher incidence of suicide. Long term medication is also an expensive practice, over many years, particularly if hospitalisation is required for acute crises.

Strangely, little or no mention is made of clinical hypnosis in the literature references and when it is, it is usually with regard to traditional hypnosis involving relaxation, self-hypnosis, bio-feedback training in hypnotic trance, progression and so on. The availability of analytical hypnosis is very rarely mentioned, except in those journals devoted to clinical hypnosis. While the professions do recognise that early traumatic experiences may contribute to Panic Disorder, they have never to my knowledge entertained the concept of the Death Expectancy Syndrome as a result of the birth experience or some similar situation.

Much research has been done on the intricate neurotransmitter interactions with various parts of the brain and body. Yet this distressing condition is a classic example of a syndrome of physiological changes which arise from an original event involving fear - be that the birth experience or some other perceived catastrophic event. Hypnosis provides the key to the road to understanding and healing.

Patient Rob

The History

Rob was a teenager with several problems, including Panic Disorder, Social Phobia, Depression and difficulty getting on with his life. He was a couple of years behind his peers ... in other words, a Ponce de Leon Syndrome.

His first sentence was:

"Well, I don't really ... I ... I don't think ... I don't actually know if there is a problem and I'm very tense and it wasn't my idea to come."

I already knew a great deal - a walking zombie doesn't know! Moreover he's 'dead' – three "don't know" phrases! I knew he was tense, he had anxiety. I knew there was some denial, which could be because of fear or embarrassment - he 'didn't want to come', which in turn alerted me to a prenatal problem and a perception of the outside world as threatening. So, his first sentence revealed a PNE, DES, WZS and PDL. Some transference was also evident - there was a hint of stubbornness. A great deal of information could be gleaned from a single, albeit long, sentence. Rob then continued, on invitation:

"I just get more anxious ... I really panic. There's more pressure as you move up. I get pressure from school. I worry about everything."

He was describing the birth experience - "more pressure as you move up"!

"I get very tense, more lethargic. I **always** have an extreme lack of energy. Short of breath. My back and arms get sore. My heart beats crazy." This was confirmation of the WZS, with the DES. On being asked, Rob said he also had headaches "all over", dizziness, numbness, diarrhoea and a nervous stomach. He had claustrophobia, and couldn't go into a situation where people had to talk to him, which is Social Phobia. His physical symptoms and panic could occur anytime, sometimes "the slightest thing triggers it off."

"I don't feel like I'm anybody or anything, it's like I'm just existing - like I'm not any particular person at all." This represented a serious Identity Problem, and with all these emotions and feelings he said he was "scared to look for things after school." I was not surprised ... this very likeable young man was in an unenviable state. For some years he had been on, and was still on, medication and had been treated by a psychiatrist and a psychologist, with no real alleviation of his symptoms.

The Word Association

DES: Anxiety = not knowing what lies outside
 Fear = alone
 Darkness = where you can't see where ... where you can't see anything.
 Cave = fear because you don't know where you can get out
 Walls = stop you from getting where you want to go
 When the walls close in = claustrophobia
 If I don't get out = I will suffocate
 My greatest fear = being alone

WZS: Live = what you can do when you're free
 I was near death when = I was two
 I became = nearly a corpse

IDP: My problem = is I don't know who I am
 Need = love
 Please = help me to be a proper person again
 It's all connected to = fear and loneliness

JDP: Sinner = me
 My greatest fault = not being worth anything
 Guilt = that I can't do better for my parents' sake
 My punishment = loneliness

PDL: I'm stuck at the age of = ten
 It all started when = I couldn't live up to expectations

I was able to now define the diagnoses and the critical events and to understand a great deal of how he thought. He had the DES, the IDP and he was a WZS: "I became? almost a corpse"! I had a good idea that this SPE was at the age of 2 years. He was also a PDL, and a SIE had probably occurred at the age of ten, when he felt he couldn't live up to expectations.

The Prenatal Experience

Rob was regressed and found himself at six months *in utero*.

T	: What do you pick up from your mother?
Rob	: Nothing.
T	: How do you feel about this?
Rob	: Sad. Alone.
T	: Is there anything you can do?
Rob	: No.
T	: Do you have sense of meaning for yourself? Any purpose?
Rob	: No.
T	: How do you regard yourself?
Rob	: Unimportant.
T	: Whose responsibility is that?
Rob	: Mine.
T	: How do you see your future?
Rob	: It doesn't seem like very much.
T	: What are you going to do?
Rob	: Just hide.

Rob was regressed further back to before and after his mother was aware of his presence - he **did** have perceptions of love then. He was then invited to go to the first time something happened that resulted in his feelings of an absence of love and reported himself to be at four months.

Rob	: Something's happened. She's worried. I'm also worried.
T	: About?
Rob	: I don't know. I'm scared. Could get hurt. I'm moving. Something could be wrong with me.

A spiritual reframing was carried out and he was requested to make contact with his younger self. However, he had a great deal of anger for the baby and this required careful restructuring until he was able to accept himself and delete the faulty suggestions he had given himself.

The Birth Experience

In the birth canal at the start of the labour:

Rob	: I'm anxious. I don't know what it is. It might be dangerous.
T	: What do you think could happen?
Rob	: I won't be warm. It might be dangerous. I could get hurt.

He needed some prodding to realise the obvious - he was avoiding the thought, the concept of death.

T	: Yes, go on.
Rob	: I won't be able to breathe.
T	: And then?
Rob	: I won't be alive.
T	: What is that?
Rob	: I'll be dead.
T	: Go on. I'm with you.
Rob	: My face is sore. I can't breathe! I can't breathe! I can't breathe! I'm gonna die!

Here his acute fear of death was followed by his own faulty suggestion that he was going to die - the WZS. He was encouraged out and helped to take his first breath, responding with the exclamation 'I'm **alive!**'

T	: Where is your mother?
Rob	: Asleep. I don't feel safe.
T	: What do you need?
Rob	: Love ... she's gone! I'll be lost!
T	: What will happen to you now?
Rob	: I can't survive! I'm going to cry until I go back. I'm hungry! But there's no-one there. Someone walked past! Something in my mouth! I'm cross because they won't take it out. I feel like I'm stuck here forever.

Rob was a victim of the Separation Anxiety Syndrome, followed by his conviction that all was lost. This suggestion had remained ever since, despite the fact that the subsequent bonding was excellent with a great deal of joy and love. These faulty beliefs were of course corrected and immediately in the next session he reported that he was much better, feeling fitter and able to concentrate. He had 'stopped worrying!' The PNE and BE were of course his ISE.

The Symptom Producing Event

As predicted by our work-up, this occurred at the age of two years. Rob apparently had a severe gastroenteritis with a high fever and dehydration and was so ill that he was taken to hospital by his parents and admitted. Rob was really 'into the swing' of regression work and described in detail how angry his anxious father was because there was a delay in his being attended to. He described how deathly ill he felt, the nurse shaving his head and the IV drip being inserted and the tepid sponge-bath to bring his fever down. He felt very scared he was going to die; his breathing was irregular until ultimately he again believed he was going to die. The straw that 'broke the camel's back' was being 'abandoned' again by his mother and father, while he was kept in the hospital! It was this event of illness which the Word Association referred to as 'I became = nearly a corpse!'

These perceptions of abandonment and death were aggravated by the arrival of his new-born sister. Naturally enough, a new-born requires more time and attention but Rob, primed with past experiences, found this traumatic. He now began to be socially withdrawn with a lack of confidence in his ability to 'simply be'.

As a walking zombie, his subconscious had to find a proof of life - his activities became increasingly directed at stimulation ... and the so-called hyperactive syndrome began with an accompanying marked learning disability and fine motor problems. Dead people don't think, can't concentrate.

This resulted in embarrassment at school with other children. Being in a special class he was marked out for ridicule which of course intensified his perception of his worthlessness and his hole in the soul. There were a couple of regressions to times of family strife between his mother and father, which increased the feelings of insecurity and his IDP and WZS intensified. He took to his bedroom and "shut my ears". He had determined to deal with all his woes in the following manner:

"I'll just stay as I am. I won't try anything, then I won't get worse. I'm scared I won't be able to handle things - I'll go crazy." Such a manner of maintaining at least one level of survival is a classic example of the Ponce de Leone Syndrome. With those beliefs which were established at the age of two (!) he simply could not interact with the world: he was stuck with the mental and fine-motor abilities of a two year old!

One significant regression in this regard involved a teacher who really 'put him down' in front of the class about his clumsiness and inability to do anything right. This was followed by his frustrated father providing the same messages. In this situation, a child is in hypnosis - such comments act as post-hypnotic suggestions: they are held as true and acted upon as true.

The Symptom Intensifying Event

Age : ten years

I encountered strong resistance to regression, whereas before there had been no problem. The cause was a perception of tremendous guilt and unworthiness which apparently had occurred in the home environment. While I was not able to elicit the dynamics, the Word Association assisted me in determining his responses - as you recall:

Sinner = me
My greatest fault = not being worth anything
Guilt = that I can't do better for my parents' sake and, (most damnably)
My punishment = loneliness

Fortunately, even though his subconscious mind was not prepared to openly discuss the dynamics, I was able to determine it was indeed a guilt problem with spiritual death and to deal with the Jurisdictional Problem subliminally ie with minimal awareness by the conscious mind - his subconscious was continuing to safeguard against potential devastating knowledge. Once this self-forgiveness had been accomplished he was at last able to freely say 'I love me' and rejoin humanity. His panic attacks resolved and his mood was elevated - he rated himself as eight out of ten, which was a fully realistic self-assessment.

We had accomplished our primary objectives – resolution of his main complaints. I believe that he will function at a higher academic level. Indeed, he wrote and passed his exams whereas before merely thinking of them precipitated anxiety. If necessary more work can be done on his PDL.

Rob demonstrates not only the development and resolution of a Panic Disorder, but also one way in which the 'Attention Deficit/Hyperactive Syndrome' – ADHD - may develop and be treated.

CHAPTER FIFTEEN

Myalgic Encephalomyelitis (ME) or Chronic Fatigue Syndrome (CFS)

This condition has other synonyms - epidemic neuromyasthenia, postviral syndrome, yuppie flu and neurasthenia. Contrary to common belief, it is not a new condition – 'neurasthenia' is a very old medical term. As a diagnosis, it has many fervent supporters and as many critics. The term 'encephalomyelitis' is misleading and inaccurate because no inflammatory process of the brain's neural tissue has ever been demonstrated. You will see that in medical hypnoanalysis there is a logical process taking place in this sometimes devastating condition.

The major characteristic of ME is primarily severe fatigue of at least six months duration, associated with significant disability and unexplained by any recognised organic disease. Numerous symptoms are present, of which eight must be present to make the diagnosis. Alternatively, just six must be present if there are two signs.

The symptoms are:

1. Muscle discomfort or myalgia (muscle pain)
2. Migratory arthralgia (pain which moves from one joint to another)
3. Generalised headaches
4. Generalised muscle weakness
5. Sleep disturbance
6. Neuropsychiatric symptoms

7. Prolonged fatigue after exercise, which previously caused little or no problem
8. Mild fever or chills
9. Recurrent sore throat
10. Painful cervical (neck) or axillary (armpit) glands
11. Rapid onset of the symptom complex

The signs are:

1. Low grade fever
2. Non-exudative pharyngitis (an inflamed throat without any pus-type material)
3. Palpable or tender cervical or axillary glands

Along with all this, there should be no psychiatric diagnosis such as a past or current Major Depression, and so on.

This condition has been the focus of a great deal of controversy in the medical fraternity and in public debate which has created considerable anger in sufferers who sought to have their very real disability recognised, lest they were all labelled as malingerers. Indeed, these patients are often persistent in their requests for further investigations in terms of blood tests, MRI scans of the brain, etc. There are of course many causes of fatigue which are easily explained in medical terms. Anaemia, low thyroid function, ordinary depression, diabetes, wasting diseases, chronic infections ... the list is long and each of these needs exclusion because they are usually easily and successfully treated.

ME certainly results in drastic changes of life-style – one need only speak to a patient to discover how their lives have been altered, and the lives of their families. The cost to the economy and health care may be significant, entailing medication for years, and costly investigations. Consider the financial implications of losing a trained and competent worker and the added cost of retraining another. Often, interpersonal relationships deteriorate which adds to the problems. They have difficulty functioning at almost every level ... they cannot work, they cannot do housework, sexual activity declines from both a lack of energy and often inclination. In terms of medical hypnoanalysis, one can already sense that they are all severe walking zombies. They are 'dead' people, the living dead.

The incidence of ME or CFS is more common in women than in men and usually occurs in young people - late teens and twenties, though this is not at all absolute. Causes put forward are varied and certainly it often follows a viral infection. The chapter on psychosomatic disease and the accompanying diagrams demonstrated that many infections follow after some emotional event, as the immune system is compromised. The most popular cause proposed is probably the Coxsackie B virus infection theory, by Yousef and his colleagues in 1988. ME patients favour this theory in particular, in my experience at least. However, while 25% of patients have antibodies for the Coxsackie B virus, a similar incidence is found in normal controls! There is also a strong seasonal variation to the condition but this is true of other conditions, including depression.

Medical treatment alone has not been found to be very helpful, except as a supportive measure and includes attention to diet, exercise, depression and so on. Adding cognitive behaviour therapy has been shown to be of greater benefit in altering patients' belief systems of the disease and the outcome. Yet many patients continue to endure its effects for two or many more years. There is often the problem, when treating these patients, of a subconscious secondary gain factor: as long as they are symptomatic, they receive recognition - be that positive or negative. Either way, this provides some positive benefit in that they have a reason to ventilate anger or receive love in its wider sense.

The fact is that there is no specific medical treatment and ME presents difficult management problems to the health care team. To one who practises medical hypnoanalysis this comes as no surprise because it has a subconscious origin in a thought (a suggestion) and an emotion.

Patient Fred

Fred was 50 years old when he came to see me and had been symptomatic for two and a half years. He had been hospitalised and treated by his company's doctor and a psychiatrist, with no improvement and had been medically 'boarded' as unfit to continue in his career. Yet he had not been to his general practitioner at all for this problem.

We went through the normal procedures ... and when asked for his full names, he left out his surname. The IDP was already a likelihood. On being asked what the problem was, he replied: "Umm" [= WZS. He then gave a big sigh = DES. This was his subconscious alerting us to his birth experience, possibly his first threat and the need to breathe]. "At the moment I'd say this sleepiness. Feeling of being giddy and a weak feeling in my knees and legs. Unable to concentrate. My sight seems to go in and out of focus. Depression that seems to come and go for no reason." Obviously, he was describing the physical characteristics of being 'dead'- the Walking Zombie Syndrome.

On being asked when this began, he said: "Definitely been building up since 1990." The accompanying event was his company moving office, a move in which he had most of the responsibility and had to endure the reactions of the senior people at work such as: "We should have done this, we should have done that." This represented a Symptom Intensifying Event. He said: "I was totally washed out." Again, this was the WZS, and a reference to his birth – "washed **out**".

I asked him if he was a worrier and he replied: "Yes, probably all my life." A very early life event was again referred to here - the PNE or birth experience. Relieving factors were "achieving something they can't do; meeting **dead**lines which are always impossible." Thus Fred had a need to prove himself to others to gain approval ... this was the PDL Syndrome, stuck with a threat to his self-esteem or mind survival. Further, he had to meet **dead**lines in order to survive. Ostensibly these were in the socio-economic area, but I was alerted to higher levels on the order of importance now - the remaining one was of spiritual survival.

His history also revealed some domestic problem between parents and grandparents, which precipitated a move of home, when he was 5 or 6 years old. His father was an autocratic, unapproachable, critical and unloving parent and he admitted to guilt feelings here. In the 8th grade at the age of 13 he had a really bad relationship with a teacher and was sick most of that year. His mother died when he was 16, leaving him 'pretty upset' - she **had** been loving.

Later in life, in business with a difficult partner who had a drinking problem he developed muscle and joint pains which were diagnosed as rheumatoid arthritis! A pattern was developing – he became ill in times of stress. This pattern had never been recognised before because **no-one** had ever taken a decent history!!

His Subconscious Diagnoses was now apparent. The ISE was probably his birth. The SIE was certainly his company's move and I had a pretty good idea of other SIEs. I was not yet sure of the SPE, but the Word Association confirmed that for me - his subconscious mind **knew!**

The Word Association
   It all started when = our first move!

And there it is: the SPE was when they moved away from his grandparents, when he was about five or six years old.

Death Expectancy Syndrome
   Fear = nothing
   At the end of the road = is a tunnel
   Darkness = nothing
   Tunnel = nothing

Associating all these, we get an expectation of nothingness, of death, and it is related to a dark tunnel.

The Walking Zombie Syndrome
   I was near death when = my mother died
   When my mother died = I lost something

What he lost of course was love and subconsciously, this is death.

The Ponce de Leon Syndrome
   As a child I = must have been pretty weak
   I became = not much better
   It's all connected to = being where I don't want to be

The Prenatal Event

This was pretty good for the most part because there was a strong perception of love from his mother. However, he felt a certain responsibility for her discomfort in being pregnant. His way of dealing with this was a decision 'to make things easy for her'. This was important because it started a pattern in which he began to put other people's needs before his own. There was also an uncertainty about the future:

T   : How do you feel about going outside?
Fred : I'd rather stay here. It's warm.
T   : Yes?
Fred : I don't know what's out there. I'm insecure about it.

The ISE: The Birth Experience

T   : What part of you is going first?
Fred : My head.
T   : How does it feel?
Fred : A bit constricted.
T   : How do you feel?
Fred : Rather tense, waiting for something to happen. It's unknown.

Fred began twitching his arms and legs and head as he abreacted his experience.

T	: What's happening now?
Fred	: There's pressure on my head and shoulders. I can't move much.
T	: How does that make you feel?
Fred	: Helpless.
T	: What are you picking up from your mother?
Fred	: She's in pain.
T	: What do you think about that?
Fred	: I'm responsible.
T	: You're not. It's not your problem. Go on now. What are you experiencing?
Fred	: I'm dizzy. I'm spinning. It's not pleasant.

Referring to his history, this was the ISE for some of the symptoms he presented with!

T	: What are you doing?
Fred	: Struggling.
T	: What do your struggles achieve?
Fred	: I'm **tired**.
T	: How do you feel?
Fred	: Scared. I want to breathe.
T	: If you can't?
Fred	: I'll drown. I'll die! I don't want to be here!
T	: Go on.
Fred	: I'm out!
T	: Take a deep breath in. Deep, deep in. Hold it there. Feel that air filling your lungs. When I ask you to let this breath out, let the oxygen flood every part of you. Let it go now! What does this breath tell you?
Fred	: I'm at peace! I'm alive!
T	: And now?
Fred	: I seem to be cut off from her. I'm a bit jittery. Insecure.

T	: Go to when you're with her.
Fred	: Ahh. Great.
T	: What is?
Fred	: Waves of joy. Love.

In the WAE, I learned, 'it's all connected to = being where I don't want to be!' He certainly did not want to be in that birth canal - that was his first brush with exhaustion and physical death and was transposed over time to when he didn't want to be in his job!

The Symptom Producing Event

T	: How old are you there?
Fred	: I'm five, or six.
T	: What's going on?
Fred	: My parents are arguing with my grandparents. It's on religion.
T	: Yes?
Fred	: My grandparents want me to go somewhere else.
T	: Do you know of God?
Fred	: Yes. I'm bewildered. I feel as if I'm the cause of it. [The argument]. I'm **in the middle.** [trapped!]
T	: How do you feel?
Fred	: Scared. My parents are cross. Unhappy. Insecure.

Again, Fred had taken on a responsibility for other people's reactions, which had to do with imposed religious beliefs. This was the precipitating factor of the family's move. Two things imprinted as a result: firstly, his father left first and it was six weeks before he again saw him - a separation experience. Secondly, he was more dramatically removed from his loving grandparents.

He then experienced another devastating separation experience - his first day at school - a Symptom Intensifying Event.

Age 7 years: First day at school

Fred : I'm feeling insecure. I don't know what is going to happen. I don't know anyone.

The unknown future had now been established as a potential survival threat.

T : Where are you?
Fred : In the classroom.
T : Where's your mother?
Fred : She left. I chased after her but she hid in a cupboard[!]
T : How do you feel?
Fred : It's the start of something new. I'm scared. Alone.
T : Anything you can do?
Fred : No. I'm helpless. I feel abandoned. Unloved. Upset.
T : What will happen?
Fred : I don't know. There's no hope. [Acceptance of death]
T : Go on now, you're home again. How does your father react to this?
Fred : He laughed.
T : What does that make you feel?
Fred : I felt worse. Embarrassed. Ashamed. I couldn't make him understand. It wasn't easy to talk to him. Stern.

Fred now had his Walking Zombie Syndrome firmly established together with a hole in the soul.

Symptom Intensifying Event 2

Age 13 years: Once again, the beginning of school - on this occasion, high school. He knew no other boys and had heard that a certain Mr Heller was to be his teacher. Fred had prior knowledge of Mr Heller through the Scout Movement and knew him to be a vindictive person.

T	: How are you feeling?
Fred	: Unhappy. Worried. Lonely. Vulnerable.
T	: Is there anything you can do to help yourself?
Fred	: No. I'm helpless. I feel trapped.
T	: I see. What is happening to your heart, then?
Fred	: It's racing. Jumping.
T	: Where was the first time you had this?
Fred	: When I was born.
T	: Yes, that's right. Go on now.
Fred	: He (Mr Heller, the teacher) sees me. He has a smile.
T	: You feel?
Fred	: Apprehensive. It's not a friendly smile.
T	: Go on. Why not?
Fred	: He came past and tapped me on the shoulder. He asks why I left his troop at scouts.
T	: Yes?
Fred	: I told him I wasn't happy with the people in his troop.
T	: What does he say?
Fred	: Nothing. Just that smile again.
T	: How do you feel?
Fred	: Fear. Helpless.
T	: Any hope?
Fred	: No.
T	: Your heart's beating. You're physically alive. What about emotionally, spiritually?
Fred	: No.
T	: It's a death-like feeling, isn't it? Like the birth canal?
Fred	: Yes.
T	: What are you going to do now to survive?
Fred	: **I was sick a lot. I stayed at home.** More than at school.
T	: You're out of that threatening environment then, aren't you?
Fred	: Yes.

T	: How does your mother respond?
Fred	: She supports me, at my side.
T	: Your father?
Fred	: He's refusing to see my side. There's no understanding. I couldn't tell him.
T	: Why not?
Fred	: I'd be ashamed. He'd reject me more. He shouted a lot.
T	: That's where it really began, isn't that so? Your illness?
Fred	: Yes. I got sick to avoid Mr Heller and school.

Symptom Intensifying Event 3

Age 16 years: when his mother died of cancer.

T	: How do you feel about her passing on?
Fred	: Sad. But relief. She suffered a lot. My father made me look after her and I didn't want to. It was painful to me. But she looked peaceful so I felt peaceful too.
T	: She's gone now. How will you cope?
Fred	: There's a loss.
T	: In terms of your own life, how do you feel?
Fred	: Dead in a way.
T	: That's right. You thought about killing yourself, didn't you?
Fred	: Yes.

Fred was now in serious trouble - it was his mother who had consistently and unconditionally provided the necessary love: a walking zombie as a result her death, it was not unusual to think of his own death, as we have discussed elsewhere. Suicide ideation occurs when one has already accepted death within.

T	: Why didn't you?

Fred   : She came to me when I was sleeping. She was all dressed in white. She tried to tell me not to worry. I felt easier. At least I didn't want to kill myself anymore.

This beautiful spiritual experience at age sixteen saved his life. I know some will say: "oh that's just his way of coping, it's imagination". I believe this spiritual energy is proof of the power of the infinite spirit.

He had a lot of suppressed anger for his father, Mr Heller and the school and was given the opportunity to understand it and give vent to it.

Symptom Intensifying Event 4

Another SIE was his business venture with an ill partner. Fred again subconsciously contrived to extricate himself from a trap: he developed 'rheumatoid arthritis' and the onset of his ME.

Age 48 years: The company was in the process of moving premises and Fred had the overall responsibility for this move.

T   : Where are you, physically now?
Fred   : In a meeting in the boardroom with consultants and three computer people.
T   : What's happening?
Fred   : No-one could make a decision how to cable the whole building.
T   : How do you feel?
Fred   : Tense. Annoyed. Tired. Helpless - it will be impossible to move on the deadline.
T   : And if you don't move by the deadline, how do you regard yourself?
Fred   : A failure.

T	: Now take these feelings and thoughts of this deadline and go back to the very first time you felt them. Go back, way back ... that's right. Where are you?
Fred	: Being born.
T	: What do you understand by this?
Fred	: I'm threatened.
T	: Yes, you're threatened. But it's not a physical threat now, is it?
Fred	: No.
T	: It's a self-esteem threat, and socio-economic, isn't it?
Fred	: Yes.
T	: How does it compare?
Fred	: As bad.
T	: What do you do? You're back with the company.
Fred	: I go to the MD. He tells me to make the decision.
T	: How do you feel then?
Fred	: OK. But tired. There's a lot of pressure.
T	: Yes, it's like that birth canal. Go on. The move is finished. How was it?
Fred	: Totally successful. But...
T	: Yes?
Fred	: The MD's attitude. He's picking up on stupid details.
T	: How do you feel?
Fred	: More and more tired and disillusioned.
T	: Who does he remind you of?
Fred	: Mr Heller and my father.
T	: What are going to do about it? What happens to you?
Fred	: Tired.
T	: What is that tiredness? What feeling is it?
Fred	: A dead feeling.
T	: That's right. That's the Walking Zombie Syndrome. What does this tiredness do for you? Does it have a purpose?

Fred	: It protects me. I don't want to be there. I don't care.
T	: Does this remind you of a previous experience?
Fred	: Yes. That's how I was being born.
T	: Right. You gave up on life then and it's become a pattern. You survive this threat. But it also stops you from living. Just like your school years and your other jobs. True or false?
Fred	: Right. That's what happened.
T	: Now, you had no choices as that baby. Do you have choices now?
Fred	: Yes.
T	: Sure you do. What choice are you going to make for **you** now? Do you need to stay dead?
Fred	: No.
T	: Is it OK to let go of these feelings, this tiredness and all the other symptoms?
Fred	: Yes.
T	: Is there any part that disagrees?
Fred	: No.
T	: Then ... let go. Now!

Fred was helped to make a decision to live and to reformulate his approach to challenges which he had previously perceived as life or death situations.

Fred realised his subconscious ploy of the tiredness: in that birth canal he had become exhausted and given up, yet survived anyway. This became a pattern of surviving other challenges in life. By his next session, he was feeling "pretty good". He rated himself at 8 out of 10 and reported his energy levels were "first class", that his motivation was high. He went back and started his own business. He grew up and became alive in every sense. His ME disappeared - for two or three years, only to return in a milder form with another Symptom Intensifying Event relating to his father's terminal illness and his **reactions** to his father's attitudes. This relapse was successfully treated with one further session.

CHAPTER SIXTEEN

Habit Disorders
Smoking, Drugs, Alcohol, Obesity

This chapter gives a general outline of the common causes of these habit disorders, the problems encountered, and their management.

Smoking

While I am greatly appreciative of my colleagues who refer smokers to me, my concern is that most doctors still believe that smoking is about the only disorder one refers a patient to a hypnotherapist for!

The tragedy is that most of these patients will not do very well, for the simple reason that they are not motivated. They arrive with the mistaken belief that this 'mumbo-jumbo' will remove the problem, and that their own efforts have no bearing on the outcome. Well, 'one can lead a horse to water but one can't make him drink!' As in the Conduct Disorders and major Personality Disorders, otherwise unpopularly known as 'psychopaths' such patients, if coerced into therapy, are a lost cause before one begins.

I have learned to ask a would-be non-smoker one question when they call for an appointment: "When do you want to stop?" If the answer is "yesterday", we get going as soon as possible. If the answer is: "well, I don't know. I thought you could do it for me", I tell them not to waste their money or my time, unless they are willing to undergo analysis. However, if genuinely motivated, the success rate is high.

Some of them require a full analysis, because there is usually an emotional reason for the smoking. To merely remove the symptom of smoking by suggestion often results in another symptom, the most common of which are weight gain and anger or irritability. The reason is simple: if we remove a symptom which to that patient's subconscious is a proof of life, the subconscious is surely going to find an alternative proof of life! If, however, the **cause** of the emotional problem is resolved, it is unusual for an alternative symptom to present itself.

A truly motivated patient can be treated in one or two sessions, most of them in five hours! I had a patient who after hypnosis and how a symptom develops were explained to him, phoned two days later to cancel his appointments. He said it made so much sense to him that he had stopped smoking already and was feeling great! As a matter of fact, a patient - friend of mine who had been hijacked twice in a couple of weeks cured himself of his anxiety in the same way - one consultation!

There are other life-long smokers who give up because the smoking - the proof of life - has now become the harbinger of death! I've known 'two pack-a-day' smokers who continued to smoke after the first heart attack and the second! However, after the third one it filters through to the subconscious that to smoke **is** to die, to not live anymore. These fellows also give up easily and wonder why they couldn't do it before. The reason is the subconscious is now faced with a greater threat - imminent and sudden physical death.

There are some smokers who **do** need an analysis even though they are very motivated. Usually, these people have not only had a prior physical death-like experience or two, (the ISE and SPE) but have also had similar spiritual death-like experiences. The following case discussion is one such patient.

Dawn - 30 years of age.

Dawn was an anxious and depressed individual. She had attempted suicide eighteen months before seeing me, and remained depressed despite adequate psychiatric treatment.

Dawn had the following to say when asked what her problem was:

"Wanting to give up smoking desperately and not having the will-power to do it on my own. My doctor told me I'll have emphysema by the time I'm 40. It started when I was eighteen, going out with friends - you have your first puff and that was it."

Wow! She had told me so **much!** She had really been wanting to **give up** on her life! With 'no will-power', she must be a walking zombie. The fact that she could not do it "on my own" indicated a Separation Anxiety, possibly Identity Problem - and certainly a Ponce de Leon Syndrome. A child needs help - not a self-supportive adult.

And the ISE? Birth of course because "**going out** with friends - you have your **first puff**, and that was it!" The first breath.

She confirmed much of this with "I don't feel myself anymore". This was both the WZS and the Identity Problem - what would be called in traditional psychology a 'depersonalisation'. "I can't get up in the morning. It's there the minute I open my eyes in the morning." The latter clearly indicated when her problem started - the birth experience. If she was cured? "I love sport, gym. **I haven't the energy, the breath!!**" She was a WZS alright and it was certainly the birth. She even blew smoke rings when younger - to the subconscious, that is being able to actually '**see** my breath - **I must** be alive!'

So I knew the Initial Sensitising Event - birth - and that something had happened before she was eighteen: which would be the Symptom Intensifying Event. This had to be some death-like experience. The history confirmed this: at seventeen she had been severely assaulted by her father, the culmination of a very abusive relationship over the years. This was the cause, to her own reasoning, for being a "nervous person - I've been a worrier all my life". This was where she had 'died' at spiritual level, and perhaps accepted a suggestion of physical death. After this event, she stayed at first with friends, then later a court-appointed foster home. Typical of a tyrant, her father told her she had been disloyal - which resulted in guilt!

What could the Symptom Producing Event be? Well, she'd had a couple of threatening situations, including a near-drowning at the age of two years.

The Word Association
   My real problem = worthless
   Depression = worthless
   The colour of my problem = black
   Black = death
   I smoke more when I'm = nervous = anxiety = fear = death
   To get rid of the fear = I need to know there'll be no more fighting.

Clearly, Dawn's problem was to do with death, and this death was perceived at physical and spiritual levels.

The Death Expectancy Syndrome:
   When the walls close in = scared
   Down in that dark hole = scared
   I've just got to = get out
   If I don't get out = I'll die
   My greatest fear = going back home [!]
   Walking Zombie Syndrome:
   At the end of the road = death
   I was near death when = I drowned

This last response indicated the Symptom Producing Event, which was where subconsciously she accepted death: she said 'I drowned' and not 'I nearly drowned!'

The Identity Problem:
   Hostility = alone
   Why = do I feel so alone
   Who = will I be one day [this also = PDL]
   I felt a failure when = I was very young

Jurisdictional Problem:
   Guilt = not being the person I'm supposed to be
   I could never do the right thing for = my father
   My punishment = hitting

The Initial Sensitising Event.

Despite having a father who appeared to be tyrannical, the prenatal experience was good. However, as we could expect from the history and Word Association, the birth experience was difficult.

Dawn	: I'm moving now, my head is going first.
T	: Good. Go on now.
Dawn	: It feels tender on the front of my head.

The first part of the birth was quite good and she was encouraged to let the time pass.

T	: Feel your heart now, what's it doing?
Dawn	: Going faster.
T	: For what reason?
Dawn	: I'm not going out much further.
T	: How does that make you feel?
Dawn	: Scared! I'm trying to get out. Unsure.
T	: If you don't move out, what do you think could happen?
Dawn	: Can't breathe.
T	: And if you can't breathe?
Dawn	: I'll die. I'm shouting.
T	: For what reason?
Dawn	: Angry! I'm not coming through ... I'm not sure I'm going to live.
T	: What else are you feeling?
Dawn	: Dizzy. Tired. Mom's pushing. Shoulders are starting to come through ... I'm **out**.

Dawn was taken through the routine of a deep breath in order for her to realise she was indeed alive. As nearly always, this breath told her "I'm **alive**!"

T	: What are you doing out there?
Dawn	: Crying!
T	: Why?
Dawn	: I'm not near my mom anymore.
T	: How does that make you feel?
Dawn	: Insecure.
T	: Without your mom, what will happen?
Dawn	: I'll die! I'm cold, and scared.
T	: Go to when she holds you. What do you feel now?
Dawn	: Warmth. **Love.**
T	: **Now** how do you feel?
Dawn	: Comfortable. Safe.
T	: Is your father there?
Dawn	: Yes. There's joy and happiness! They're taking me away now! I'm feeling **lost.** Crying. Sad ... worried.
T	: Where do they take you?
Dawn	: To a room.
T	: How do you feel there?
Dawn	: Alone.
T	: What is it you're frightened of?
Dawn	: I won't live.

This, then, was the ISE for her anxiety and the compulsion to breathe. It was the cause of her physical WZS as she accepted the idea that she may not get out of the birth canal **and** the cause of the Spiritual WZS with the removal of love. The separation anxiety was clear, followed by a loss of hope - hence her depression. This experience again indicates the dynamics of anxiety usually preceding a depression period, or co-existing with it: first a fear of not surviving, then the loss of hope and acceptance of death.

The Symptom Producing Event

Age 2 years - near drowning

T   : Where are you?
Dawn   : Out in the country. We're having a picnic. There's lots of people. We're going to have lunch but I'm not at the blanket.
T   : Where are you?
Dawn   : Running down towards the water. Mom and dad don't see me. They're not taking notice.
T   : Go on.
Dawn   : I'm looking at the bottom of the water. I jump in.
T   : Go on. What happens?
Dawn   : I'm going down. Frightened.
T   : Yes, Dawn, you're frightened. For what reason?
Dawn   : I'm going to die!
T   : What are you doing? [She was very agitated as she abreacted]
Dawn   : I'm fighting and kicking. Breathing getting less. Filling up with water. I'm going further down. Starting to lose energy. I'm drifting. I'm fighting. I've reached the bottom. Almost no energy. Lungs are engulfed with water. Head very heavy. White. I'm very still. I'm lying at the bottom. Heart slower.
T   : What are you thinking?
Dawn   : I am really dying. Still frightened. I don't seem to have much feeling left.
T   : Go on. What happens?
Dawn   : Feels like someone lifting me now. I'm lifting with a big speed.
T   : Yes?
Dawn   : It feels like I'm on something hard now. Someone shaking me. I hear lots of noise. Someone is putting their mouth over my ... it feels good ... water coming up ... I'm coughing ...

T	: What does that mean to you? To cough?
Dawn	: I'm starting to get air in my lungs.
T	: Yes?
Dawn	: I'm breathing.
T	: And if you're breathing?
Dawn	: I'm alive!
T	: So as long as you cough, you're alive?
Dawn	: Yes!
T	: Go on now.
Dawn	: I see my father. He's crying. I feel sad for him but happy I'm starting to breathe. He's pushing down on my chest.
T	: Take a **deep,** deep breath in and hold it. Hold it. Now slowly let it out ... good ... what does that breath tell you?
Dawn	: **I'm alive!** Everyone ... lots of laughter and happiness ... I feel wonderful. Still coughing a bit.
T	: That's fine. When you've coughed enough, let your yes finger tell me. Good. Now, you **know** you're alive. You didn't die. You **thought** you did, but you didn't. I want to ask subconscious, do you still need to cough to know you're alive?
Dawn	: No!

In cognitive therapy in trance we were now able to establish that the coughing was a proof of life - her subconscious contrived to produce a great deal of mucous in her lungs to **make** her cough.

Dawn	: As long as I coughed I knew I was alive!
T	: What was the purpose of the smoking then?
Dawn	: It made me cough!
T	: When was the **first** time you had to cough to be alive?
Dawn	: When I was born!

Very significantly, as a result of this experience she saw her father as the single reason she was still alive - his subsequent behaviour could therefore not be challenged! Particularly with the commandment 'honour thy father and mother'.

The Symptom Intensifying Event

There were a series of these, all contributing towards a sense of uselessness, bad self-image and hopelessness. All of them were related to her father.

Her word association indicated her sense of failure – 'I failed when = I was very young'. This was intensified at the age of thirteen when she had a bad school report - father beat her, leaving marks on her arms. She felt unwanted, rejected, and unloved - she developed a hole in her soul, and began to **believe** that she herself was inherently bad. By the time she was fifteen years old, the situation had deteriorated so much that she had given up all hope of appeasing her father. Her mother was powerless to intervene, as were her siblings. She began to lose hope for her future - it was no longer worthwhile, not with the situation at home. She became a true walking zombie.

The First Cigarette: Age Sixteen

T	:	Where are you?
Dawn	:	With my best friend. I feel good there.
T	:	For what reason?
Dawn	:	I'm not at home. There's nothing to worry about here. We're by the pool. She asks if I've ever tried [smoking]. I tried. Made me feel very dizzy. Not good initially. I carried on, more puffs. Better. Getting used to it. Calm.
T	:	What makes you calm?
Dawn	:	Being with a friend, smoking with her. It's more belonging. I don't belong at home.

T	: So it's more 'belonging' that you need, isn't it? And the smoking? What does that do for you?
Dawn	: I breathe in deeply.
T	: Yes?
Dawn	: Importance. It makes me feel alive.
T	: Dawn, do you feel like that at home?
Dawn	: No! **Not** at home.

Thus a conditioning of smoking to induce calmness was initiated. It wasn't the cigarette *per se,* but the companionship, the acceptance, the **escape** from home - metaphorically, **getting out** of the threatening birth canal, out of the water ... having the space to breathe! Dawn associated the physical act of breathing in cigarette smoke with the emotional gain of acceptance. The severe beating at age seventeen was a further SIE, in which she was so physically damaged that she accepted death once more. It also resulted in the intensification of her spiritual death.

One last fear needed to be removed, and this was to do with a major guilt problem - the JDP, the details of which I choose to withhold. Accept from me that she went through an experience in which she blamed herself intensely for an alleged 'wrong'. The truth was that in order to survive what she felt was a greater threat, she had no choice. When she understood all the prior conditioning which had preceded this event, she was able to forgive herself, thereby removing the last obstacle, because part of her self-punishment included the ill-health.

This achieved, she stopped smoking just like that. Snap!

Obesity

Obesity ... volumes have been written about it, thousands of research projects have been undertaken and little has changed in the perceptions of its origin and treatment. Once more, it is consigned to the genetic code pile by most. An editorial by ARP Walker in the *SA Medical Journal* succinctly reviews what we know and what we don't know, informing us that obesity costs Americans 33 billion dollars a year on weight control efforts, also that the State pays a further seventy billion dollars in respect of health economics. He describes these figures as 'staggering'. One hundred billion dollars a year – and this was 1999! I wonder how many primary health care programs around the world that would pay for? While sixteen percent of women in the United Kingdom are considered obese, forty-five percent of black South Africans fall into this category. I wonder why? I believe apartheid had something to do with it; separated families and therefore poor support systems - rejection and repression because of the colour of one's skin. One could go on and on about the South African scenario but what I wish to emphasize is that those policies were SPEs and SIEs.

Obesity is an extremely common disorder, and is being recognised more and more by the health professions as a disease. But what type of disease - physical or emotional?

A study published in the *Journal of Child Psychology and Psychiatry* examined the role of self-esteem in its relationship to body weight. The conclusion was that there is "no clear impact of overweight on children's self-esteem". While this may be surprising to some, it is no surprise to a therapist. As mentioned elsewhere in this book, the more successful a symptom is, the less emotional residual there will be: it is the primary goal of the symptom to reduce the anxiety, fear or guilt! However, such research and the one hundred million dollar industry deflect attention from the real causes, over and above genetic predisposition.

The following short case graphically indicates the negative effects of religion presented in a manipulative manner, according to the perceptions of the child. It also demonstrates another interesting medical phenomenon: the belief that certain prescribed drugs have unwanted side-effects.

Side-effects of drugs are common but it has always intrigued me that some people endure feeling awful while others on the same drug don't 'turn a hair'. Why should this be? No-one can provide answers to this question, except to say it is an idiosyncratic (a personal quirk) happening, probably on the basis of one's genetic make-up.

This patient, a Catholic, became very overweight in her adult life, having previously had a good figure. Indeed, she related the onset of her obesity directly to taking the contraceptive pill. The real reason she gained weight was later apparent. She had spent a great deal of money on trying to lose this weight. She saw her own doctor, tried all kinds of diets and consulted two experts on obesity.

Of the latter she said that she did indeed lose weight but put it all back on and more stating **"It was all my fault,** because I didn't follow the maintenance diet". By now, I **knew** she had a guilt problem - the JDP. Her Word Association confirmed this:

My punishment = to suffer!
When I die = I'm going to suffer

Diet. The word itself conveys to the subconscious the threat it is under: **Die…**t. Bad word. Bad practice. Consider if the subconscious has provided this symptom to maintain life and one attacks this symptom, one can expect some resistance. As many fat people know, this is exactly what occurs. One can certainly lose weight by sustained starvation (which is what dieting is) but nearly always, this weight is regained with some insurance added. The next time the patient diets, it becomes more difficult to lose the weight and it takes longer to do so - the metabolism is altering, favouring weight conservation. So it is not only that fat people eat more, they alter their metabolism which makes it difficult to lose the weight. Ultimately, some of these people develop what is called 'refractory' obesity - another word for resistance.

Her Regressions - Patient June
The Initial Sensitising Event: age 4 years

June	: I'm with my mother at a bus stop.
T	: Right. How are you feeling?
June	: Horrible.
T	: For what reason?
June	: She's shouting at me. She's found some pencils in my case - they aren't mine.

T	: How did they get there, June?
June	: I don't remember.
T	: What is she saying?
June	: She's going to punish me. She's going to tell my teacher. God is going to punish me!
T	: If she tells your teacher, what will happen?
June	: She'll punish me. She always hits me.
T	: Always? Go to such a time. You're right there. What's happening?

June went to her Symptom Producing Event:

June	: She's hitting me.
T	: How do you feel?
June	: Horrible. I'm scared of her.
T	: For what reason?
June	: She's a nun.
T	: What does her being a nun mean to you?
June	: She's God's representative.
T	: So what does that mean to you?
June	: God is punishing me! I'm bad.

Symptom Producing Event: age 28 years

June had recently had a baby and as there was a financial crisis at home, she had to return to work and could not afford to fall pregnant again in the foreseeable future.

T	: Where are you, June?
June	: At the gynaecologist. He is giving me the pill.
T	: How do you feel?
June	: Horrible. Guilty. He won't put the loop in.
T	: What does being on the pill mean to you?

June	: It causes abortion!! But I'll have to take it.
T	: What do you think God will do about this?
June	: He's going to punish me!
T	: How?
June	: He'll send something terrible to happen to me. I'm scared.
T	: What are you going to do about this?
June	: I'll have to be strong.
T	: What happens to your appetite?
June	: It's good.
T	: And your body?
June	: It gets bigger.
T	: Look at your body, June. How does it look?
June	: Horrible!
T	: And how does that make you feel?
June	: Horrible! Worse!
T	: And you're feeling horrible inside. It's like your body is matching how you feel. Let subconscious tell me, does this fat serve a purpose then?
June	: To make me horrible.
T	: Is this a punishment?
June	: Yes.

The problem of obesity is therefore not a problem of medication, it is not a problem of calories or kilo-joules, it is a problem of **survival!** Usually, this survival is at the spiritual level. I must emphasize that not all fat people have guilt as the cause: anxiety and fear are not uncommon.

June had been indoctrinated as a child to fear God. The threat of his punishment was used to steer her away from unacceptable social behaviour. Whether or not she stole those pencils is irrelevant - this is a classic example of how religion is used as a manipulative weapon by usually well-intentioned parents and other authority figures. Her fear of God was reinforced by her nun teacher and she totally accepted the suggestion that she was indeed a sinner, and that punishment was now inevitable come Judgement Day. This highly charged suggestion remained in the subconscious, waiting for a trigger. She had also learned the faulty idea that the 'pill' causes abortion. This is not true - it prevents ovulation, so no fertilised egg or fetus ever develops.

As 'artificial' contraception is a sin in Catholicism, she was doomed to guilt in her Catch-22 position as a mother who **had** to work. She was able to understand that it wasn't her mother who punished her, or God. It was indeed herself - she had acted as prosecutor, judge and executioner in fear of Divine punishment to come … she pre-empted her expected punishment by God at some future time in the hope of lenience. She had to **suffer**: the Jurisdictional Problem.

Fat people do suffer: socially, sexually, in their self-esteem, in their health, with high blood pressure and all its eventual effects, diabetes, and so on. They begin to sacrifice at economic levels too. Note that all these symptoms occur at all levels below spiritual on the Order of Importance. Survival at the level of God's love and the continuation of the spirit are paramount, superseding all other needs of survival.

Taking the contraceptive pill had absolutely no bearing on her fat problem. Gaining weight was purely a psychological mechanism, mediated through various physiological processes and not the hormones in the pill, which is a smaller dose than that provided by the body.

Her appetite centre was stimulated. A neurotransmitter called leptin was no longer produced in her body, or a great deal less than normal. Leptin sends the message to the hypothalamus in the brain 'hold up! We have enough fat stores now!' Even while she ate more, her body utilised energy far more efficiently! Many people believe that in obesity, the body's metabolism is less efficient: this is not true. In order to promote fat storage, it is **more** efficient.

Like a bear storing fat for the winter hibernation, the subconscious is compelled to provide for an expected threat in the future. This is why our patient June became fat - she was not only punishing herself, she was protecting herself. She had decided; she had the thought that she must be **stronger**. That thought was translated subconsciously - she **was** getting stronger!

She was getting bigger. This protection and punishment were no longer necessary for her to survive and she subsequently, steadily lost weight.

CHAPTER SEVENTEEN

Cocaine Addiction

All people suffering from chemical addiction have one thing in common - they are dead inside. This may be a Walking Zombie Syndrome at physical level but nearly always they are also Spiritual Walking Zombies. Usually there is a significant Jurisdictional Problem and an Identity Problem as well: the latter is what sets them up for the spiritual death.

The chemical addictions are not easy to treat and it is essential that these patients have a genuine desire to be well. Very often, they pay 'lip service', and agree to treatment because of pressure from their families, or employers, or problems with the law. However, they have no real intention of changing. This applies to alcoholism, cannabis, heroin, amphetamines or cocaine addiction and of course, the problem is often multi-drug abuse. Another difficulty is to prevent further drug use whilst under treatment. A session may bring to the surface a great deal of pain, which some patients try to alleviate by 'bingeing', cancelling out much of the good learned during therapy. Continued drugging or drinking delays healing, and I will not treat anyone who is not at least temporarily free of his chemical of addiction.

My own addiction experience taught me that once I had made my real decision, to live, it was a lot easier than I expected it to be. The axiom of each and every day was quite simply: "The most important factor, the priority, of my life is not to use pethidine again. I don't need it. There are alternatives. Like ... **living**".

Patient Eric

Eric was thirty-two when he consulted me. His history was very typical of severe addiction : he was about to lose his job, was not coping with his work, felt isolated from people and very, very depressed. He had financial problems. More typical, from a medical hypnoanalysis point of view, were his first few remarks in the history. He omitted his surname when asked for his full names, indicating that he probably had an IDP.

"The only time I feel is when I'm rushing - when I'm snorting coke. Empty, apathetic. The so-called emptiness varies in degree but I suppose it's been there about twenty years."

This was a typical description of the Walking Zombie Syndrome: the only time he **felt** was when he snorted coke, otherwise, he was dead! His cocaine snorting was very clearly his proof of life. Since he described a physical **feeling,** I knew his real problem was higher up in the order of importance - at mind or spiritual level. Emptiness and apathy typified a dead state as well - and he provided me with a possible time of a significant event, about twenty years ago.

Asked what aggravated the problem, he said: "Having to get up in the morning". I guess the average doctor or psychologist cannot be blamed for an inward sigh and the thought "Oh here we go again with the usual cop-out. This guy's got no prognosis. I can't work with him." Tragically, that is not an uncommon response. I knew a colleague, who quite bluntly refused to see any alcoholics in his practice. What these doctors are missing, apart from a degree of humanity, is that the patient is actually telling them what the problem really is and when it began!!

Eric couldn't get up in the morning - he did not want to face the light of day or the world. His problem was either in the prenatal experience or birth, or **both!** That was where he had first 'died'! Simplistic, yet it is true! So I knew the Initial Sensitising Event!

The Symptom Intensifying Event was probably 'about twenty years ago'. What happened to Eric? At the age of thirteen, he and two of his friends were walking home from a soccer match when a taxi mounted the pavement and struck them. One friend was killed. Eric was severely injured with head trauma and lost consciousness! This tragedy was a reasonable cause for the WZS.

Eric told me quite a bit in the first five minutes of his history - he told me about the anger he used to have as a child. He then volunteered, without being asked, that "I think what triggered the tantrums was my folks were going out and I didn't want them to - something like that." I was to discover that this incident was part of his Symptom Producing Event.

Eric also told me that as a child in primary school he was a rebel, which had resulted in problems in the family and at school. This behaviour would today have been diagnosed as 'Conduct Disorder' - a precursor to an antisocial personality. How quick we are to judge, and with such ignorance!

The Word Association
   My problem = me
   God = me [!]

That is, his problem was **God**! So, I was dealing with a Jurisdictional Problem at the very least. This was confirmed as we continued, because although he said 'when I die I'm going to ... Heaven', he later said:

When I die, I'm scared I'm really going to = hell!
I sinned when = I killed my friend
My punishment = life!
Guilt = always! [always? ...]
Sinner = coke

Death Expectancy Syndrome
   Darkness = fear
   My greatest fear = death
   Down in that dark hole = death
   When the walls close in = suffocate
   Breathe = wheeze
   Asthma = breathe

My deepest thoughts tell me = I'm scared
How = does one get out of here

The Walking Zombie Syndrome

I was near death when = (Sigh) [=DES], every morning, every night
Instead of snorting I'd rather be = breathing
Death = life
This was an important response, because when associated with 'my greatest fear = death' I knew he was fearful of life! No wonder he had trouble getting up in the morning!
When my friend died = I shut myself off
My greatest desire = death [!]

So not only was 'doing' coke a proof of life, but his behaviour was killing him as well - the ultimate punishment and the ultimate escape from his pain.

Rushing lets me know = I'm alive
When I snort = warmth, real
Without coke I = don't exist

The Identity Problem

My problem got worse when = I realised I was alone
When I give up = I want to be real
To lead a normal life I need = to find myself
My mother never = loved me
My father never = loved me
If I had been a girl = often wondered about that
I'll be able to stop when = I'm real

The Ponce de Leon Syndrome

As a child I = fucked up
I became = even more fucked up

The Initial Sensitising Event: The Prenatal Experience

Eric regressed initially to four months *in utero*.

T	: How are you feeling there?
Eric	: Alone. Sad.
T	: For what reason?
Eric	: They're fighting.
T	: How does that make you feel?
Eric	: Separated. Like I'm an interloper. I don't belong here.
T	: Are you picking up on any love?
Eric	: There's no love.
T	: What do you think about that?
Eric	: I'm not loveable.
T	: Do you feel any purpose?
Eric	: No.
T	: Any meaning?
Eric	: No.
T	: Do you feel responsible for her?
Eric	: Not responsible. But exacerbating her problems. Guilt. If I wasn't here, she'd be better off.
T	: What are you going to do?
Eric	: Die. It's easier, warmer.
T	: Does she reject you?
Eric	: No.
T	: Who rejects you?
Eric	: God. I feel like two entities. One which is me, passive. Other part dead.

Eric was taken further back, to before his mother was aware of the pregnancy. There, not yet two months, he became aware of warmth, of a light. He became aware of a certain peacefulness and was able to realise that the subsequent problems he felt, the judgements he made were based not on his genetic code but rather on his limited knowledge and his perceptions of other people's problems - that they were nothing to do with him. He regained a sense of meaning, an acceptance of God in his life and was able to assist his smaller self in these understandings, as if **he** as an adult, was the caretaker of this hapless fetus. Disaster turned to hope, the emptiness of death turned to life - spiritual meaning, unconditional acceptance, love.

The Birth Experience

Now a Spiritual Walking Zombie with an Identity Problem, the birth began.

Eric : I'm moving now, my head is going first. Very strange. Worried.
T : About?
Eric : My head feels like mush. Skew. Painful.
T : What do you think about this?
Eric : My head's going to pop. It's giving me no room. I feel constricted – my chest and my throat.
T : How are you feeling?
Eric : Panic. Big panic. Something choking me - I'll die. Trying to breathe. Can't breathe. Scream. Struggling. Just the overwhelming feeling – to breathe. Someone, something's taking the pressure from my throat. I'm out.

Eric took his first breath with the response: "I'm alive!"

T : How do you feel away from your mother?
Eric : Scared! I'm screaming with relief and anger. I want my mommy!

T	: Go on.
Eric	: I wee!
T	: What does that tell you?
Eric	: I'm alive! I can breathe and I can piss! Let me enjoy this! … With my mother.
T	: Good. What do you pick up from her?
Eric	: Warm. Relief. Joy. Hatred.
T	: What's the hatred about?
Eric	: With me, I think. Ambivalent. It's not me.
T	: What about love?
Eric	: I'm not too sure. Upset. My mom's been squashed. My fault.
T	: How do you feel?
Eric	: Guilty and scared that I won't be able to breathe. My chest and throat are sore.
T	: Where are you now?
Eric	: Cold green room. No-one there.
T	: What is going to happen to you?
Eric	: I don't know. Don't know if I can make it.
T	: Go on. Let time pass.
Eric	: Surrounded by people now. My family.
T	: What do you pick up from them?
Eric	: Angry. My mother's angry.
T	: Who with?
Eric	: Me, I think. It's OK because my gran is holding me … she wanted a girl.
T	: How does that make you feel?
Eric	: Confused. Like a part of me is missing. It's almost as if a part of me died - in the womb. Guilty.
T	: For what?
Eric	: I don't know. I just feel I'm to blame.

So Eric's Death Expectancy Syndrome had begun, as had the Walking Zombie Syndrome, at a physical level. The JDP of guilt became entrenched and his vulnerability without love, his loss of unconditional acceptance, the IDP, intensified. It is important to note once more that these were his very profound **perceptions**. From a practical point of view, whatever the reality of the situation was, these impressions resulted in an already set pattern of emotional and cognitive responses - even behavioural responses. It's why he'd wondered about whether he should be a girl. The birth experience was the cause of his asthma, and his anger. He **needed** to **hear** and **feel** himself breathing to know he was alive!

Symptom Producing Events

    a) Age five years

T	: What's happening?
Eric	: Confused. I don't fit in. My brother is sick - they didn't tell me!
T	: How do you feel about that?
Eric	: Ostracised, alone. There's less love from him now.
T	: Where are you getting love from?
Eric	: My dog.
T	: Your dog?
Eric	: My mother doesn't let me in. Doesn't let me in.
T	: What about your dad?
Eric	: Nebulous. There, but never there. No hugs. He's nice to my friends, not to me.
T	: And how does that make you feel?
Eric	: Alienated.
T	: Go to when something happened, that you became rebellious.
Eric	: I'm seven or eight.

T	: Go on. What are you doing?
Eric	: Drinking his brandy.
T	: For what reason?
Eric	: I did it to rebel.
T	: How did that make you feel?
Eric	: As if I was **there**. Someone noticed me! He smacks me. My dad, everyone is angry except my gran - she loved me. I had to look in the mirror while he hit me with his belt.
T	: What does that pain tell you?
Eric	: I never cried.
T	: Why not?
Eric	: Angry. I was a non-entity. They couldn't be bothered. My brother was sick. I felt guilty about him being sick. I should have understood. Wish they had let me be a support.
T	: What did you do?
Eric	: I slept out a lot. Very angry.

b) Age seven years

T	: Where are you?
Eric	: At home. My brothers are there.
T	: Your parents?
Eric	: They're going to see a movie.
T	: How are you feeling?
Eric	: Scared. I'm feeling deserted. I'm very angry.
T	: What is their reaction?
Eric	: Mother's laughing. I feel useless. Like I'm not there.
T	: Take these feelings way back now, way back to the very first time you ever felt them. Right, you're there. Where are you?
Eric	: In the womb.
T	: What is it you're scared of?

Eric : I'll die.
T : That's right Eric, but you did not die. You are alive. Come back now to seven years. Your father - how does he react?
Eric : He wants to go.
T : What are you thinking?
Eric : I might have to stay. Helpless. Scared. Angry! I want to break things. Crying uncontrollably.
T : What do you do?
Eric : I just crawled back into myself.

Eric had 'died' again – life just did not matter anymore, he was depressed. His behaviour deteriorated even further. As no-one really understood his need - love - this was met with anger and disapproval which alienated him even more.

Eric was basically a very fine human being, with a huge potential for loving, but very few people recognised this, least of all himself. Tragically, he had already judged himself on past alleged failures, as being unworthy of being a part of the family. He did not believe he deserved success in life.

The Symptom Intensifying Event

Age thirteen years

T : Where are you?
Eric : We're walking home from a soccer match we went to see. We left at half-time.
T : Go on. Who's with you?
Eric : My two friends. There's no pavement - we're walking almost crabwise. I squeeze myself between them.
T : Go on.
Eric : We turned the corner. I hear brakes ... a squeal. It turns into a scream.

T : Who is screaming?
Eric : It's me. I got sore - my head.

Eric became very agitated now - writhing.

T : What's happened, Eric?
Eric : My friend's bloody and squashed.
T : What are you feeling?
Eric : Pain. Loneliness. Colours - just red.
T : How do you feel?
Eric : It's my fault.
T : For what reason is it your fault, Eric?
Eric : Because I convinced the guys to watch a movie. I can't look. I can't see. There's blood in my eyes. It's like blacking out.
T : What is happening to you with this blacking out?
Eric : Dying. Pain. Screaming. I vaguely remember an ambulance. He's really squashed. I can't speak.
T : What has happened to him?
Eric : He's dead. I can't speak. Like everything is blank. It's my fault!
T : It is not your fault, Eric. Go on!
Eric : I'm drowning in blood. Fighting. It seems ages. Red, mangled bones. It's like I'm flowing in this tube. If I let go I'll drown.
T : Eric, I'm going to count to three and you'll be in the hospital. One, two three! Describe where you are now.
Eric : In a strange bed. Tubes sticking into me. Arm, hurts. My brother is there.
T : Yes. Go on.
Eric : He says my friend is dead.
T : What do you feel?
Eric : Horror. It **is** my fault.
T : What are you going to do about all these feelings, Eric?

Eric   : Shut everything out.
T   : How does that help?
Eric   : Can't think. Can't feel.
T   : Can't feel what, Eric?
Eric   : The guilt. Can't speak. Like a block of wood in my mouth.

[Eric did not speak for two months after the accident]

T   : That's right. It helped you, Eric. It was too great a burden at the time. Feel your own heart beating. Physically do you feel alive?
Eric   : Yes. I dissociated! [Spontaneous realisation]
T   : That's right. Emotionally, do you feel alive?
Eric   : No. I want to die!
T   : Spiritually?
Eric   : No.
T   : Where is God, then?
Eric   : He can't exist.

Based on his childhood concept of God as a watchful old man in the sky, Eric had to deny the existence of God - firstly to avoid divine punishment and secondly to rationalise this tragic event.

This denial was intensified when a few months later another friend, with malicious intent, said to him: "It was your fault!" Having denied a deity, he no longer felt guilt - he simply could not afford this human 'luxury' and survive. The price was to become a walking zombie – 'dead' at both physical and spiritual levels. He had already accepted his own death physically and as part of the Jurisdictional Problem, had to punish himself - he 'wanted to die.'

T   : What happened to you afterwards, Eric?
Eric   : I became introspective. Had nightmares.
T   : About what?

Eric	: The crash. My friend. I screamed in my nightmares.

[Indeed, Eric had Post-traumatic Stress Disorder]

T	: What else happened, Eric?
Eric	: I became a real brat.
T	: That's right - your behaviour got worse. How did that make you feel, being a brat?
Eric	: Alive [!]
T	: What did you do about the nightmares?
Eric	: Dope. I couldn't sleep with the nightmares.

And so began his behaviour disorder and his career of drug addiction. Cannabis eliminated the spiritual pain. Cocaine, a powerful stimulant – and it was exciting - gave him a sense of being alive. Recall the Word Association – "Rushing lets me know I'm alive" and "Without coke, I don't exist". It also provided his punishment: again, from the Word Association, "My punishment = life" and later: "death = life!" That is to say, his punishment was death. As his drugging continued, he certainly suffered. It was in fact slowly killing him, which was his subconscious wish.

A good person, and he **is** just that, he was created in innocence and purity, but he never believed it of himself and could not believe it, **only as a result of his life's perceptions,** a prisoner of his own perceptions from way back in the womb. This negative conditioning very nearly destroyed him. He had never believed himself to be 'real', to have any rightful place in this world, a reject in life. Remember the word association –'to lead a normal life, I need to = find myself.'

A very careful restructuring of his guilt was successfully undertaken, though this was neither easy nor straight-forward. His Identity Problem was addressed, his inherent spirituality was rekindled, reinforced and accepted. **He had to accept himself -** to say "I love me". There was no other way that he could arrive at that point without understanding his origins by regression. He was then provided the opportunity to choose to live - which he did, eliminating his Walking Zombie Syndrome.

Eric displayed a courage that is quite remarkable. His story is my tribute to him. It says a lot for the human spirit and the potential we all harbour.

CHAPTER EIGHTEEN

Personality Disorder

There are several different types of personality disorder, ranging from the fairly benign to the worst kind of Antisocial or Dis-social Personalities. This last group includes the popular term 'psychopath'. The milder non-aggressive types include Obsessive-Compulsive, Anxious or Avoidant and Dependent personality disorders. The Obsessive-Compulsive type is discussed in the next chapter. This chapter looks at the more legally significant dis-social type, a group that tends to become involved in criminal activities and generally in behaviour which is unacceptable to society.

In 1993, Girolama and Reich published an epidemiological study of this problem under the auspices of the World Health Organisation. The incidence varies around the world: from 0.1% in a survey in Taiwan to 9.8% in a midtown Manhattan study in 1963. Generally, between five and ten percent of the population have a personality disorder!! I would venture that in South Africa today, this figure is a great deal higher, which is not surprising, if one considers the forced separation of children from their parents by the pass laws and the general philosophy of apartheid. The developing violent culture would have exacerbated the problem and I believe contributed to the inevitable self-destruction of apartheid as an ideology.

The sequences of events and perceptions of the patient in the previous chapter are very typical of the development of a Conduct or Personality Disorder. Eric did not become a Dis-social Personality Disorder - he was not able to suppress the guilt sufficiently. A personality disorder he **did** indeed have, but a lesser one. The reader will now begin to appreciate my dislike for formal diagnostic labels in isolation. They are perhaps necessary in the greater scheme of things, but they do not assist the patient.

The following statement will no doubt also be considered controversial. Each and every one of the personality disorders has a cause, a **treatable** cause, though this was not consistently the case until the philosophies of medical hypnoanalysis were applied. Perhaps the worst aspect of diagnostic labels is that they categorise and often condemn people. Most therapists avoid the personality disorders like the plague, only, I contend, because of ignorance.

The Dis-social Personality (DP) arises because of a perception of death, especially spiritual death: the removal, actual or perceived, of love. This spiritual death is accompanied or soon followed by, the perception of physical death. These perceptions are the result of a prior event - the ISE - usually in the PNE or birth experience. This event is perceived as overwhelmingly threatening to survival. After fearfully and unsuccessfully exploring all alternative avenues of escape, the individual absolutely accepts his own death as a protective defence mechanism against further assault, which is considered by the subconscious to be potentially catastrophic to further functioning.

To continue the struggle for survival would result in overwhelming, unbearable and unacceptable 'pain'. To 'die' is the ultimate protection, because by being 'dead' the pain can no longer be experienced. In effect, the individual permanently shuts out the threat so that it no longer need be endured. This defence **persists** as a protective device thereafter. He cannot allow himself to again be hurt by a similar threat.

This type of individual becomes what I term an 'Absolute Walking Zombie'. Of interest is that when these patients are asked in regression at the point of this death acceptance if they still feel fearful, they answer "No, it's OK now!"

With the idea of being 'dead', activities now begin to focus on stimulation-seeking behaviour which provides the proof of life. Being dead at spiritual and mind level, this behaviour is directed at the remaining levels of the order of importance: physical, socio-economic and sexual. These patients, so condemned and rejected by society, 'simply' have a different agenda, a different set of priorities.

This single-minded pursuit of the proof of life results in the 'abnormal' behaviour - their subconscious priorities are different, alien to society's rules. Being 'dead' they cannot again be hurt at conscious level, and this knowledge is self-reinforcing. In childhood, 'naughty' behaviour develops and is an attempt to gain some attention, **any** attention: They are saying "Hey! Someone please see my pain! **I need love!**" The behaviour certainly achieves a proof of life, as does the punishment. These children discover that the physical pain of punishment is over quickly, that it does no long term damage. In fact, the pain itself is a physical reminder of life. They learn that emotionally they cannot be further harmed because they have switched off so much. This revelation brings a sense of **power** and power is life, along with the anger of injustice. An endless cycle is set up which is self-reinforcing. The punishments serve another purpose - atonement for the faulty self-imposed guilt they feel. Ultimately, even the guilt is switched off. It has become too threatening to their spiritual survival.

Coercing or punishing these individuals may strengthen the defence by subconsciously recreating the original threatening environment of abandonment, anxiety, fear and guilt, with no recourse to outside help or understanding. All manoeuvres become acceptable in the pursuit of proof of life. Emotional barriers such as guilt do not apply if one is 'dead'. Lying and manipulation become tools to avoid further pain - they become weapons, not restraints. A family with such an individual is an unhappy family. Interpersonal relationships are devastated.

Being 'dead' they are unable to provide love, they cannot maintain a relationship: it's a one-way street. The corollary is also true - it is difficult for someone else to maintain a relationship with them. There is a secondary gain for these patients in their limited relationships - they are protected against another rejection or separation experience. They have difficulty in having any sustained emotion.

The text books describe these patients as under-aroused and **bored**. This is because they are dead - boredom and death are subconsciously synonymous for them. They **must** be stimulated, so they begin to seek dangerous, or at least exciting, physical activities - they need the rush of adrenalin. They may be sexually promiscuous, and they may be very successful in business, or for that matter, in any sphere where they can gain power - the military, politics, even in religion. One has only to review some of the publicised activities of some 'churches' to see the light. It is an extremely disturbing thought that many of the world's leaders have been, are, and **will be** Dis-social Personality Disorders. They achieve success because they have no remorse. What drives them is their need for power, to feel alive.

Being 'dead' it is not possible to learn from experience, because it is the experience itself which is important, not the learning. There is no necessity to learn - they are locked into an immature pattern: the PDL Syndrome. To learn would mean to lose their only way of maintaining some level of life. There is a rather frightening fatalism in these patients.

Most health professionals shudder when presented with such a patient. Many avoid them, considering them a waste of time and effort. It is not uncommon for a family with such an individual to be told: "There's nothing we can do - you'll have to learn to live with it".

There are professionals of course, who do not abandon their patients, or clients. The Robert Wood Johnson Medical School in the USA has a program in which they treat and educate the parents to manage their 'Conduct Disorder' children. They have found that "most commonly we see children with conduct disorder coming from families where there is violent, abusive behaviour; alcohol or depression. These problems have persisted for a number of generations." The question is: are these conditions inherited, or a process of conditioning? A child who has not been taught to love him- or herself cannot consistently provide love to others and their children will perpetuate the problem. While genetics may play a part, the fact that these people **can** be assisted favours the origin as being largely negative conditioning.

The Robert Wood Johnson Medical School's program is expensive - about 5000 dollars per parent as at 1999! Well, I have two colleagues who treat the **children,** as young as four or five years of age, with great success utilising medical hypnoanalysis, at about a fortieth of the cost! These children often require only four or five sessions, as there is less to work through and the results are simply wonderful, which certainly provides food for thought.

Conduct Disorder and Dis-social Personality Disorder patients are certainly treatable, especially when the results of their behaviour have led to conditions worse than the ISE, the original threatening event eg, when they are facing a long term in jail: incarceration traps them, recreating the original event of their 'death'. Subconsciously, these patients are now more open to therapy.

Patient Sam

Eighteen years old, Sam was brought to see me because he had been arrested for an alleged theft and was due to appear in court. He had had a 'behaviour problem' for some years, and was often in trouble with authority. He had escaped the wrath of the law before due to technical matters and sheer luck. Note the minimising of his problem – 'behavioural': no-one would even confront the family with the truth.

His history was characterised by the following information from his father:

He was always in trouble at school and was a "rebel", the "class clown". He was easily bored and did "not follow through". Expelled from school in the tenth grade, he disliked authority and usually confronted these people with anger. At one time he had set fire to school property in a rebellious gesture. He was very manipulative and had one arrest for drunken driving. His mother was described as "highly strung" and was quite ill during the pregnancy. The birth had been two weeks late and was difficult, with the cord around the neck. When Sam was six years old, his mother had simply absconded and left the family.

His first three sentences:

"This is hard to say. [It is, for a dead person!] I think when my mother left I took the attitude 'well, who cares a damn'. That deteriorated into an attitude of not caring for the consequences of my actions. I started going out a lot, smoking and drinking."

Asked when this began, he said "Pretty much after the initial shock. I was never able to express my feelings. I've always ... well, always since my mother left, been like this."

Asked what made him feel better, he replied: "Nothing. It's not a bad feeling - I live with it. I'll probably land up dead or in prison. I'm sure it won't be a favourable outcome. I just realise I've got to stop."

Sam was brutally frank and his last admission indicated that his behaviour was subconscious - consciously he realised where his actions were taking him, but he was unable to effect a change. He didn't want to because he felt OK with it!

The Word Association

Very commonly and almost diagnostic were the repeated responses of "nothing", indicative of the WZS.

My problem = don't know = when I was born
It all started when = my mother left

Death Expectancy Syndrome
Fear = no fear
Anxiety = no
My greatest fear = death

These patients often deny anxiety and this is logical: there is no anxiety when you are already 'dead'.

Walking Zombie Syndrome

Death = my mother
I was near death when = my mother left
Depression = mother [= dead!]
I became = depressed [= mother = dead]
Life = nothing

Identity Problem
    My mental picture of myself = nothing
    My childhood = nothing
    Who = am I

Jurisdictional Problem
    Guilt = nothing [= life]
    My punishment = nothing
    My reward = nothing
    I sinned when = dishonest
    It's so easy to = lie
    My greatest fault = dishonest = steal
    [Note the denial of guilt - he cannot afford it, yet admits to dishonesty]

There was another response typical of DP:
    When = I get older, I'll be rich.

This confirmed that he **must** function at socio-economic level, because he was dead at physical, mind and spiritual levels.

The Prenatal Experience

Sam regressed to seven months *in utero*.

T	: What are you picking up from your mother?
Sam	: Nothing.
T	: How do you feel about that?
Sam	: Scared. Lonely. She's anxious.
T	: Are you aware of any love?
Sam	: No.
T	: How does that affect you?
Sam	: Bad. Empty. Like dying inside.
T	: Do you feel any purpose, any meaning?

Sam	: No.
T	: What do you think about the outside, your future?
Sam	: Not good. Don't want to go.

As has been found in many other cases, this was the reason for the delay in labour – he was not comfortable to contend with the outside world. In the PNE, Sam had accepted spiritual death.

The Birth Experience

Sam	: There's something wrong. There's something round my neck.
T	: How do you feel?
Sam	: Scared.
T	: For what reason?
Sam	: I could die. Can't move. Pain for my mother.
T	: What does that mean to you?
Sam	: Worried for her. Will cause her distress.
T	: And if she has enough distress? If something happens to her?
Sam	: I'll die!

At the best of times a baby's instinctive knowledge is that mother is essential for its own survival. Here, Sam had this belief powerfully and lastingly intensified; when his mother left this had catastrophic consequences for him.

T	: Go on. How does your heart feel?
Sam	: Beating fast. Struggling to get out.
T	: What emotion causes this struggle?
Sam	: Anger. Can't get out. But the more I struggle, it gets tighter round my neck. Panicky. Tired.
T	: Do you have any hope?
Sam	: No. It's no good.

Sam now accepted physical death and the seed of the WZS was sown.

Sam : I'm out!
T : Take a deep breath ...

[It was apparent that he couldn't - he was choking in abreaction.]

Go on, what's happening?

Sam : [After some gasping] Can't breathe! Going to die! [breathes now]
T : That's right, take a **deep** breath now - hold it, hold. Hold it there. Feel that air filling your lungs. Let it out now. Good. What does this breath tell you?
Sam : I'm alive!
T : Right! You are alive. What happened there?
Sam : Something was blocking my throat. [the cord]
T : Yes. But it's gone now. You can breathe and you are alive. How are you feeling there now?
Sam : Too bright.
T : Where's your mother?
Sam : Don't know!
T : How do you feel about that?
Sam : Bad. Worry.

Sam experienced a separation anxiety when he was taken to the nursery - he felt abandoned, vulnerable and responded with anger until he gave up and slept. The repeated sequence of fear, anger and surrender was significant. When eventually returned to his mother, she had ambivalent feelings towards him. His perception was that perhaps he had no place there at all, that **he** was the problem.

By this stage then, Sam had already developed the IDP, the DES, the spiritual and physical WZS and a dose of the guilt of the JDP. He had a belief that his life was dependent on the presence of his mother: he also had the Separation Anxiety Syndrome and had begun a response pattern of anger and giving up when he felt matters were beyond his control. He had already found that 'giving up' eliminated the fear.

The Symptom Producing Event

A couple of significant events followed which intensified his physical and spiritual sense of fear, anger and surrender. One of these was his tonsillectomy at the age of four, when he was held down because he struggled against the suffocating sensation of the mask. Another was his mother's attitude towards him. Apparently she ignored him in pursuing her own needs. His angry temper tantrums in seeking attention were completely ignored. He was filled with a sense of loneliness and helplessness, progressing to hopelessness.

The Symptom Intensifying Event – 6 years

Sam	: I'm at home. My mother has gone.
T	: How do you feel about that?
Sam	: It doesn't bother me. I don't care anymore. Maybe it was because of me.
T	: What do you think of yourself?
Sam	: Bad. Otherwise she would have stayed.
T	: Is there anything that helps you? Your father?
Sam	: He's more worried about himself. I'm angry! It's unfair.
T	: Does that help? The anger?
Sam	: A little. But he's cross with me when I shout.
T	: And?
Sam	: I'm angrier. I just carry on. I don't care anymore. It's my problem now.
T	: If you didn't have this anger, what would be left?
Sam	: Nothing.

T   : What are you going to do about this feeling of being bad?
Sam   : I ignore it.

Sam had learned, tragically and too early, that life was his own responsibility and, mistakenly, that communication was pointless. He was carrying out this behaviour of defiance to preserve his own self, not expecting any assistance from his parents. As an infant his mother had represented life or death to him and with her gone, he considered himself as good as dead.

There was no longer meaning to his life, except a subconscious compulsion to **feel** alive. Since the feeling of guilt in this endeavour hampered this compulsion, he had simply deleted it. His behaviour became progressively "naughty" and of course, was responded to with anger from the authority figures of both his father and the school. He found that when given canings, the pain stimulated him - he felt alive! At the same time, he had a significant realisation at an emotional level: "They can't hurt me anymore!" This realisation empowered him.

His expulsion from school was not a negative experience at all. In fact, it removed him from an environment where he felt threatened - as important an escape as his birth.

However, inside he was experiencing the pain of an abandoned six-year old child, or more pertinently, the pain of a much younger child. He needed love, and there was none for him. This inner child was hidden from the world and protected.

Increasingly, he also found that his habits, the smoking, drinking and 'misbehaving' provided a sense of being alive - they excited and adrenalised him.

By the time he reached eighteen, stealing some item from a shop was part of this challenge, the proof of life. When he was apprehended, he had no real feelings:

Sam   : I'm not frightened. I think it's going to be bad - jail - but it doesn't worry me. It should, but it doesn't.
T   : Are there no feelings?

Sam	: No, I don't care. It's dead. Can't feel.
T	: Is there a purpose to this switching off?
Sam	: Yes. It protects me. It's embarrassing for the family. Not for me.
T	: Did you know what you were doing?
Sam	: Yes. I just didn't think of what might happen.
T	: How did it feel, stealing?
Sam	: Exciting. Alive!
T	: Are you feeling any guilty feelings?
Sam	: No. Only afterwards, in my room. Thinking. He [father] is angry with me. Disappointed in me. There is a gap between us.
T	: How did that arise?
Sam	: I created it.
T	: For what purpose?
Sam	: To protect myself. I don't think he ever really understood.

Sam still had a long way to go, but he was able to recognise that his immediate reactions to situations - anger, impulsivity - were the reactions of his childhood. He had a difficult time, but he changed. Most importantly, he allowed himself to feel again, to love. He was careful about this, choosing whom he would love - but this was responsible behaviour, as well as protective. The point is he is no longer dead. He has a good prognosis, and he fulfils his potential today. Like the cocaine addict, Sam is basically a good person. We all are ... from the very beginning.

CHAPTER NINETEEN

Obsessive Compulsive Disorder (OCD)

OCD is the fourth most common 'mental' disorder and presents in a variety of ways. Its incidence is increasing and one reason for this, according to various journals and proceedings of symposia, is a relative 'loss of stroking, touching behaviour'. Again, this euphemism must be correctly read as a loss of **love.** It is time we confronted the real issues and became unashamed of talking about love.

There are four essential characteristics to OCD. The patient is firstly involved in a repetitive compulsive thought and action. Action always follows a prior thought, but the thought may be a subconscious one. The patient is also aware that this thought or action is not 'normal' - that it is pathological. Next, the patient feels compelled to carry out this thought and/or action although number four, he or she consciously does not want to comply with the compulsion. Failure to do so, though, results in that person becoming very uncomfortable - an anxious agitated state. The compulsion **must** then, perforce, be a **subconscious imperative** - a survival directive.

Thus, a person on parking and locking his car feels compelled to check that the doors are indeed locked. He may walk around the car several times testing each door handle. He recognises this as bizarre behaviour, is not very pleased by it, is embarrassed by it, but can do nothing to stop it. He may be ridiculed by his wife, girl friend or friends, which adds to his discomfort. He may even go on to other disorders such as avoidance behaviours, social phobias. Other examples of OCD are kleptomania, compulsive eating, gambling, self-mutilation, rituals of washing and many others.

These patients are full of doubts and fears ... they have the Death Expectancy Syndrome. Remember that ultimately, all anxiety is a fear of death. This anxiety represents this fear when there is no obvious survival threat in the present. The basis of the threat that most OCD patients perceive subconsciously is that of a loss of love - the Identity Problem, a threat to spiritual survival.

They may also have the Jurisdictional Problem, especially those who are mutilating themselves with cigarette burns and the like. The Ponce de Leon Syndrome is obvious because they are arrested at a particular behaviour learned at an earlier age. Fifty percent of OCDs present before the age of fifteen and this is only after a Symptom Intensifying Event. The ISE and SPE of course take place earlier.

Recent evidence indicates we are closer to identifying the biochemical dysfunction: glutamate is a perpetrator, not in excessive amounts, but rather when the serotonin levels at the neural junctions are inadequate. So it does not help to restrict glutamate - this is like restricting sugar in hyperactive children. One must aim at increasing the available serotonin which can be effectively achieved with antidepressant drugs in the majority of these patients. Here again, we must ask the question "what has caused the drop in available serotonin - a wholly genetic phenomenon? Or ..." Let us examine a case history.

Patient Wyn

Wyn was thirty years old when she came to see me with the following story:

"Doctor, it's difficult to say - I have a problem with money. [giggles]. I have this idea I must always have money with me and I will contrive any way to do it. I know in myself it's wrong - terribly wrong, but I go on. It's like I can't control myself."

She described to me how anxious she became when she had these compulsions and how very guilty and ashamed she felt as this had caused tremendous financial difficulties for the family: her OCD was largely that of compulsive spending. Fortunately, she has a very understanding and loving husband who was prepared to help rather than abandon her.

In her first four sentences, she had described what took me the preceding paragraphs in this chapter to explain. What else was she telling me? Well, she left out her surname when asked for her full names, so there was probably an IDP. Looking at the first three sentences:

"It's difficult to say" was the WZS - dead people find it very difficult to speak! Her giggling about this very serious problem, which she herself had recognised, indicated childish responses: the PDL Syndrome. "I have this idea I must **always** have money with me" – 'always' indicated the PNE and birth experiences for the ISE. Finally, there was significant guilt to deal with - the JDP. The giggling in spite of her serious problem indicated a childish reaction – the PDL syndrome. The Symptom Producing Event probably took place in childhood, an assumption I could make because of her giggling. The Symptom Intensifying Event? I asked her when it began, and she replied "I was 19 - when I began to work. I spent my whole salary on myself."

Her history revealed several significant death-like situations: a near-drowning, her tonsillectomy, her father leaving at the age of two years, being sent to live with her grandmother when her mother married again, a sexual molestation, boarding school. People have responded to this kind of story with the comment, "so what, others have had it worse". Believe me, when all this happens to a child under the age of nine years, it is an unmitigated disaster for that child.

The Word Association.

Death Expectancy Syndrome
    Darkness = fear = tunnel
    Fear = when I was 8
    I just have to = get out
    If I don't get out = I'll die

I'm afraid when = I'm alone
When I'm afraid = I take money

That is, "I take money when I'm alone because I'm afraid and my age was 8 years! What I'm afraid of is dying".

Identity Problem
    Wyn = don't know
    My father always = made me scared
    My father never = cared
    My mother always = was absent
    Death = pain in my heart
    When I was born = it was a mistake

Jurisdictional Problem
    When I die I'm scared I'm going to = hell
    Guilt = pain
    Pain = between my legs
    My punishment = pain [= between my legs = in my heart = death]

Ponce de Leon Syndrome
    As a child I = had a wish to grow up
    It all began when = after my mother got married

Here was a tragic picture of an abandoned terrified child who, after being molested, believed she deserved to die. Her OCD of spending money which she did not have relieved her anxiety and was the proof of life, while at the same time punishing her.

The Prenatal Experience - Five months *in utero* :

Wyn   : She doesn't want me.
T   : How do you feel, then?
Wyn   : Rejected. I wish I wasn't here. I wish I could go away. I want to be dead.

Seven months *in utero* :

T	: What do you pick up from your mother?
Wyn	: Nothing.
T	: Any love?
Wyn	: Empty.
T	: What colour would you give this?
Wyn	: Dark. Like dead.
T	: Go on.
Wyn	: She's divorced already. A lot of pain ... and alone. She's scared and unsure.
T	: How do you feel?
Wyn	: Also scared. Alone.
T	: Is there anything you can do?
Wyn	: Go away into the emptiness.
T	: Do you feel any meaning or purpose for yourself?
Wyn	: No.
T	: How do you feel about yourself?
Wyn	: Bad. I blame myself.
T	: For what reason, Wyn?
Wyn	: She'd be better off without me.
T	: Do you have any hope?
Wyn	: No.
T	: What do you think of the outside?
Wyn	: Uh uh. Don't want to go.

Wyn had a marked experience of rejection and the faulty beliefs that she was worthless and the cause of her mother's problems; that she had no reason to be alive. Her defence mechanism was to withdraw, to dissociate herself emotionally from these feelings. She had accepted her own spiritual death after a great deal of anxiety.

A very careful reframing of her value as a child of God was carried out in which she was able to accept this truth - that her very existence had nothing to do with the choices of her parents: they were merely the vehicle for her being. She was able to utilise her understanding and reasoning to accept herself as having a rightful place in the universe and in God's love. She was assisted in letting go of the faulty beliefs and replacing them with love, truth and hope. A radical change had begun.

The Birth Experience

This followed the usual pattern of pressure, feeling trapped, increasing fear, anger and struggle, tiredness, helplessness, hopelessness and eventually an acceptance of physical death: the DES and the WZS. The immediate postnatal period was also threatening with separation from her mother:

Wyn : Unsure. Not safe. Worried.
T : What about?
Wyn : I'm not sure what is going to happen to me.

Several events occurred early in life which served as Symptom Producing and Intensifying Events for her depression: firstly, her father left her mother when she was two years old. This was a significant abandonment.

T : How old are you?
Wyn : Two.
T : What's happening?
Wyn : My father has left.
T : How do you feel about this?
Wyn : He doesn't love me.
T : What kind of feeling is that to you?
Wyn : Black. Dead.

Her mother remarried when she was six years old. This was a man who drank to excess and physically assaulted her mother, leaving Wyn utterly vulnerable and fearful of the worst, that is, death. She regressed to an event at eight years of age - the word association said "fear = when I was eight!" Her mother unjustly accused her of a wrongdoing and abandoned her - told her she would have to go. This eight year old packed her bags, phoned her grandmother and went to stay there!

The SIE for her depression occurred at nine years of age when she was sexually molested by her stepfather, an event she dared not tell anyone about for fear of further rejection and spiritual death, as a result of which she developed the full blown JDP of guilt. She was later to punish herself with period pains with her first menstruation, a rejection of her womanhood.

The Symptom Producing Event

She was now 'set up' for her obsessive behaviour: alone in the world, in fear of every moment, she was sent to boarding school at nine years of age.

T	: Where are you?
Wyn	: At the post office. I want to phone my mother. I miss her.
T	: Go on.
Wyn	: She answers the phone, but I don't have enough money. She can't hear me. [Wyn had *no money* to put into the pay phone!]
T	: How do you feel?
Wyn	: A pain in my heart.
T	: Do you have any hope?
Wyn	: No.
T	: What do you do?
Wyn	: Just give up.
T	: What colour would you give this feeling?
Wyn	: Black.
T	: What is this feeling, this colour?

Wyn : Death. It's like I'm dead.
T : So, you don't have enough money to speak to her. If you could speak to her, how would you feel?
Wyn : Better. Closer. Not dead.
T : What does this now mean to you, to not have enough money?
Wyn : I must have money, otherwise ... there's nothing.

The Symptom Intensifying Event

T : How old are you?
Wyn : Eighteen.
T : Where are you? What is happening?
Wyn : I've got my first pay cheque.
T : How do you feel?
Wyn : Wonderful. Secure. Excited.
T : And how does that make you **feel?**
Wyn : Alive. Not dead.
T : What do you do?
Wyn : I spend it. On clothes.
T : And how do you feel about this?
Wyn : Wonderful! I don't have to be scared now.
T : What if you didn't have money?
Wyn : Dead.

Money was now established as the proof of life - she simply **had** to have money to spend - it excited her, it made her feel alive. She had to have money as much as she needed to breathe. Since she had accepted physical 'breathing' death before, her proof of life had to focus on socio-economic factors: money. This spiritual and physical WZS was resolved and the need for money began to dissipate. She felt more and more in control of her life. At the last follow-up, this obsession with money and the compulsion to spend it had disappeared altogether.

CHAPTER TWENTY

Cancer

Much has been written about cancer, its causes and effects and phenomenal research continues into this disease, which for more and more people is less of a scourge, no longer a death sentence. With early detection, more effective therapies and a more positive mindset, there is no doubt that cancer **can** be beaten - even the worst kind. For example, I have a friend who had a malignant melanoma removed and was well for a decade until he had a recurrence in his lymph glands. He was not deterred and after further surgery, chemotherapy and a little hypnosis four years later is **well.** He is perfectly healthy. The key to survival in this patient is his positive outlook - he never doubted his future, and lives in the present.

In addition to all the valuable and essential scientific knowledge, we are also gaining insight into the mind and how it affects cancer. Two doctors well experienced in this field are Drs Simonton and Bernie Siegel, both of whom have written hallmark books on the subject and continue to help their patients with, and beyond, medical science. Bernie Siegel calls this and other conditions a 'reset button' - like some beacon demanding attention for change, **if** that patient is prepared to do so. Norman Cousins' book *Head First* has contributed greatly to our knowledge on this subject.

It is becoming apparent that many cancer patients - and I am not saying all patients - experienced a significant event one to two years prior to the onset of the cancer. This is being recognised now by surgeons who previously had no cause to. This prior event corresponds to the Symptom Producing or Intensifying Event in medical hypnoanalysis. That is to say, an emotional or spiritual trigger occurs. This event is sometimes not initially recognised by the patient as significant - indeed it is often denied, but nevertheless, it does occur.

It is said that in order for a cancer to develop, three factors need to be operative: a genetic predisposition, a toxin and ... an emotional gate. As mentioned in an earlier chapter, the expression of a gene may be altered by stress. Toxins can certainly be identified and eliminated, and today in many patients we can effectively deal with the emotional gate that opens to allow the cancer to develop. We can close that gate - the future is a great deal brighter than before.

The following patient is such an example. In her early middle age, at the time of the first consultation, she was confused because the surgeon had told her she was going to die, yet years later, on chemotherapy, she was still alive. She felt herself to be "in a corner - I can't go without chemo and the chemo is killing me. Most of the time I feel like "**I'm in a corner and there's no way out.**" Obviously, she was telling me that the birth canal was significant to her disease!

Patient Meg

She did not give her surname when asked for her full names, so there was probably an IDP too.

The First Three Sentences

"**Whew**! That's difficult. I'm **suffering** from cancer. I **went through** a very big operation and the doctor gave me six months to live. I'm on chemotherapy and now it's taking its mental toll. That's one of the reasons I'm coming, is to handle it if it goes on and on." Asked if she was a worrier, she replied "Oh yes, **Always**. I've **been through** depressions in my life."

What could be gleaned from the gifts her subconscious offered? Well, "Whew" was an expression of breathing - her first response, and indicated the birth experience with the Birth Anoxia Syndrome. "That's difficult" was an indication of the WZS - dead people find it difficult to do anything, and the difficulty itself is a proof of life. "I've been through" again indicated the birth and she repeated these words shortly afterwards. A critical examination of her statement "that's one of the reasons I'm coming, is to handle it if it goes on and on", revealed that this really meant "I've already accepted my own death and I need help with my suffering." This suffering was as much a burden of the soul as it was physical and indicated guilt. Her use of the word "always", was fairly indicative of the ISE: PNE and/or the birth experience.

She had had her operation - a colectomy, in which part of the colon was removed - five years previously and had also undergone radiotherapy and chemotherapy. On follow-up nearly three years later, a mass was detected in the pelvis for which she had further radiotherapy and chemotherapy, the latter for the past two years. At the time of her analysis, she was still on it. The mass did not change a great deal with this therapy. In fact, she said. "I know it's there, I can feel it."

I asked her if there were any related events around the time of her cancer diagnosis and she replied that she had gone back to university to study ... two years before the diagnosis was made!

She said: "They really expected a lot from us and I've driven myself terribly. You know, I **had** to get a distinction. I had to do everything perfectly. I really think I've driven myself too much." This of course, not only provided the SIE but also something of the underlying psychodynamics. She was obsessed with proving herself to be the best she could possibly be, despite her family's distress about how hard she pushed herself. The question was, when and why did this become necessary for her survival?

Furthermore, the recurrence of her cancer, which necessitated her current long-term chemotherapy, coincided with her elderly mother moving in with her. Her sisters had refused to accommodate her.

Her medical history did not include a near drowning - she consciously could not remember such an incident in the history. Yet, during one of the early sessions she had a spontaneous regression to a near drowning when she was very young. She had a tonsillectomy before going to school. Her family life was not good at all. She was terrified of her mother and was sent to live with her much older sister at the age of three years. She was exposed to the concept of church and sin at an early age in her religious upbringing.

The Word Association Exercise

The Identity Problem
    My real problem = myself
    Basically = I don't know who I am
    Without love = cannot exist
    My mother = never cared about me
    Underneath it all = deep hurting = rejection = when I was born!

The Death Expectancy Syndrome
    The emotion of my cancer = fear
    Fear = blackness
    Death = blackness
    My greatest fear = to die

The Walking Zombie Syndrome
    My mental picture of myself = black = death
    Please = let me live

The Jurisdictional Problem
    My greatest fault = in myself
    When I die I'm scared I'm really going to = hell
    Guilt = for what I have done to myself
    My punishment = to suffer

So it was obvious that cancer = death. Since she could not exist without love, her illness represented that death - conforming her body to the emotional image. She had judged and sentenced herself to that suffering.

The Symptom Producing Event?
    It all started when = I was small

I did not need to elucidate this further. Her subconscious mind obviously knew what the real problem was and we would get to it in due course.

The Initial Sensitising Event

The ISE for spiritual death - IDP and spiritual WZS - was in the prenatal experience: she regressed to three months *in utero,* with her mother's awareness of her presence.

T	: What are you picking up from her?
Meg	: She's glad, but also upset.
T	: How do you feel about this?
Meg	: Terrible. She's upset about having a child.
T	: What do you think about this?
Meg	: She doesn't want me ... I won't be born ... I'll die.
T	: What colour do you give these feelings?
Meg	: Black.
T	: How do you feel about yourself?
Meg	: I'm nothing.
T	: You can feel your own heart beating - physically, do you feel alive?
Meg	: Yes.
T	: Emotionally?
Meg	: No.
T	: Spiritually?
Meg	: No.
T	: Are you aware of any meaning or purpose for yourself?
Meg	: No.
T	: What do you feel about your future?
Meg	: Not very hopeful.
T	: Meg, how are you going to protect yourself from all this?

Meg	: I'll die [!]
T	: How will that help you?
Meg	: I won't feel.

The Birth Experience

T	: How do the contractions feel to you?
Meg	: Traumatic.
T	: What part of you is going first?
Meg	: My head.
T	: How does it feel?
Meg	: Just scared.
T	: Of?
Meg	: Just not to go through with this. Feel suffocating. Scared. Can't breathe very well.
T	: If you can't?
Meg	: I'll die.
T	: Is that the reason for your fear?
Meg	: Yes. I can't move my arms. Powerless.
T	: Do you have any hope?
Meg	: No ... given up. I think maybe I'm not going to make it. I've got stuck. Can't breathe. My head is burning. It's getting crushed. I think I'm through.

Meg was provided the opportunity to take a deep breath and to realise she had in fact survived.

T	: How do you feel now?
Meg	: It's light. Cold. I'm crying.
T	: For what reason?
Meg	: I think I don't want to be there. Very lonely.
T	: What is it you need right now?
Meg	: Someone to hold me. They wrap me.

T	: Where do they take you?
Meg	: I don't know, but not to my mother.
T	: Go to that time you're first with her. What do you pick up?
Meg	: No warmth. No love.
T	: What does this tell you?
Meg	: She's rejecting me. I don't want to be there.

Meg had decided to 'die' while still in the womb. As a new born, her situation was even worse because at least she was warm and relatively safe in the womb. Outside she was more vulnerable. She felt no reason to live and this intensified her desire to die - simply to survive her pain. There was literally nothing she could do.

The Symptom Producing Event

The SIE was actually a series of death-like experiences, both physical and spiritual, **when she was small**, as indicated by her subconscious in the Word Association. Firstly, her perception was that her mother was unhappy all the time - clearly depressed. This allowed Meg to continue to feel lonely and scared.

The arrival of her sister when she was three years old resulted in further isolation – in fact, she felt sorry for her sister! The tonsillectomy was a physical death experience for her:

Meg	: They've got the mask on my face ... struggling ... they're holding me down [theatre staff, take note!] ... terrible smell ... like death ... can't breathe ... they're cruel.
Meg	: What do you feel is happening to you?
Meg	: I'm going to die ... going grey. [Into anaesthesia]
T	: What's happened?
Meg	: It's like death.

Again she was allowed to realise that she had indeed survived the surgery and anaesthetic. However, this time her response was: "I just wanted to die."

The other physical death experience - the Walking Zombie Syndrome - occurred with the near-drowning:

Meg : Terrible feeling I'm going to die ... water over my head ... this feeling I'm dying ... can't breathe ... water in ... sinking ... I think I died there.

However, the real Symptom Producing Event for her obsessive need to be good occurred as a three- year old, when she was sent to live with her older sister - her mother now being occupied with the new baby. This was not a bad thing for Meg as she was happy to be away from her mother. Indeed, she dreaded her mother's visits: "She's dressed in black ... ominous ... she's just angry. [I feel] scared, hopeless."

Though far better off at her sister's home all was not wonderful:

Meg : It's much better ... she loves me ... but I don't belong there either.
T : For what reason, Meg?
Meg : She's expecting her own baby ... I'm like an intruder. I **have to be good**. There's no unconditional love.

Meg learned to perform to others' expectations of her in order to be accepted, never mind to be loved. She **had** to be good to survive. This thought established the Ponce de Leon Syndrome and later in life, this behaviour resurfaced with tragic consequences - in a manner of speaking, this was obsessive-compulsive behaviour. Meanwhile, back at her sister's home:

Meg : I had to go back to my mother. My sister felt I should go back because she had her own baby. It feels terrible. I'm scared.

Meg perceived another powerful rejection here; whether it was real or not, she **felt** it.

T	: How do you see your future now?
Meg	: There's no hope for the future.
T	: How do you feel about yourself?
Meg	: All this greyness around me ... I want to die.
T	: But you don't die, do you, Meg. How are you going to survive this? What do you decide on?
Meg	: **I try to be a good girl. I just go into myself** and live in my own world. I feel different. There's something wrong with me. Very sad.
T	: Do you like yourself?
Meg	: No ... because I'm different.

Meg therefore became dissociated, embarking on a behaviour of approval seeking, and disapproval avoidance. It was of great importance that around this time she experienced another, greater threat - indeed, the last straw. Prior to the above experiences, she had drawn great comfort from the knowledge of God's love. To a great extent this inner strength had helped her to survive. She had a belief in a very loving and personal God. However, at the age of five years, this strength was jeopardised:

Meg	: There's a lot of preaching about hell and sins. That frightens me.
T	: What frightens you?
Meg	: This powerful God and going to hell.
T	: What do you expect could happen there?
Meg	: I'll suffer.
T	: What's happened to the God you knew?
Meg	: That was a different God.
T	: Do you talk to anyone about this?
Meg	: I'm too small to verbalise.

The logic available to a five year old in abstract philosophical thinking is minimal. Such a child is likely to absolutely believe what she has been 'taught' and imprint a negative belief system - at the very least a very confused belief system which leaves her vulnerable.

T : How are you going to avoid this 'new' God?
Meg : Be **good!**
T : And if you're not so-called good?
Meg : I'll be rejected by God.
T : How are you going to be good in this way?
Meg : Helping others.

The picture was beginning to emerge, the chain of events which intensified these faulty beliefs. Meg became quite obsessed with religion when she was a teenager. This followed the wholly unnecessary and damaging guilt which resulted from masturbation.

Meg : I just feel bad about myself. I'm going on religious camps, just freak out on religion ... It's not enough, it doesn't help me. There's no escape.
T : Escape from what?
Meg : **This void that I'm in.** There's no human love. And I'm frightened of losing His love.

I have little doubt that if Meg had had a genetic predisposition to schizophrenia, this is what would have occurred. We now were ready to explore the dynamics of the body-mind in terms of the cancer. By the age of seventeen, conditions had deteriorated.

T : What is happening?
Meg : I'm rejecting my body ... got a sort of hate for my body ... it's not what I want ... it's overweight.
T : What was the purpose for the overweight?
Meg : To make me stronger ... because I felt like nothing.

T : Go on.
Meg : I'm driving it, to achieve things. Forcing it to do things, to do better and better.
T : What goal do you have for this?
Meg : My self-image will be better. For recognition from other people. I think they despise me.
T : Go on, now. To the time when the cancer had its origins.
Meg : I'm studying. Driving myself more than ever before.
T : Yes, you told me you **had** to get distinctions. Without distinctions, what do you expect will be the result?
Meg : It's life or death. My husband thinks it's totally unnecessary, but I can't help it - it's survival.
T : Go back to where this survival need first occurred.
Meg : It's at my sister, I'm small and I have to be good.
T : That's right. Now you're at university again.
Meg : I'm always so tense. Unbearable. I'm doing very well.
T : What does your body say?
Meg : I'm actually going over the limits. I know I'm hurting my body. I never let myself relax - I know I'm harming my body. I know it's wrong. But my mind and my body are separate. **I feel guilty.**
T : If you don't continue this driving?
Meg : I'll fail. **I will be nothing again!** Tight feeling in my stomach all the time.
T : What is it telling you?
Meg : That something is going to happen to me. It'll make me stop. And I'm not paying attention to those warnings.
T : Go to the critical time now.
Meg : Still studying but now there's something wrong with my body. Pain. I go to the doctors. They give me medication ... then I'm realising I've got cancer, I know it. His face is very serious. His whole expression tells me I'm going to die.
T : How do you feel?

Meg	: Shocked. Confused ... it's just so terrible. I can't go home after this ... I can't tell my husband - I know it'll hurt him so much. Feeling guilty because I know I did it to myself.

Meg was assisted further with the realisation that there were reasons for 'doing it to herself' - reasons to do with survival and punishment, both of which were now obsolete - they were the result of the survival reasoning of a three year old. She reworked her guilt and finally made the decision to **live.**

T	: Is there any further purpose for the cancer?
Meg	: No.
T	: Is there **any** part which still requires the cancer?
Meg	: No.
T	: That's right. It's purpose has been served and today you are stronger than ever before. In every way. It was there to stop your obsession, which had it continued would have destroyed you. And it was also punishing you because of guilt - a guilt you never should have had and which in any event is now **gone**. You **are** alive and you can now make that choice, can't you? Let me ask subconscious, is it now **OK** to **choose** to survive?
Meg	: Yes. Now that I'm alive and at peace, it can go!

This decision was then undertaken with the assistance of various hypnotic procedures.

Meg's therapy was not yet over, nor was the analysis. We then proceeded into several sessions which involved rehabilitation and reinforcement. We metaphorically removed all the negatives of her life and reconstructed a new life. We empowered her inner mind, and her conscious mind. She changed. However, it was apparent she was not yet at peace within.

She was asked to return to the time of the recurrence of the cancer and in this regression she again felt pain; then to return to the event which was the cause of the recurrence.

Meg : My mother is moving in. I don't really want her to but I can't do anything else. I have to carry the burden.

T : What emotion is present?

Meg : Anger! With my sisters, because they refused. Maybe angry with myself as well. Because I can't refuse - I feel sorry for her.

T : What do you do with this anger?

Meg : I suppress it because it doesn't help with my sisters.

T : Where does this anger go?

Meg : My stomach, I think.

T : How do you feel?

Meg : Trapped. I feel guilty all the time. If I go somewhere and do something nice she says "I'll be all alone again." Now I feel obligated.

Meg was able to relate these emotions to when she lived with her sister where she felt she was intruding, and to the prenatal experience. We confirmed the pain had to do with her anger and guilt and that her escape was to 'sleep' - figuratively and literally. Figuratively because eventually her cancer would provide the ultimate escape ... the sleep of death ... but not before suffering the discomfort of pain and the chemotherapy effects.

Suffering in this life is often utilised by the subconscious with the hope that if I suffer enough now I will be spared by God.

It was significant that in her first three sentences she said "it goes on and on", ie her painful, poor interpersonal relationships with the family were going ... on and on!

After two years of chemotherapy in which no significant change had occurred, her next MRI scan revealed the following: "A tiny soft tissue mass is seen in relation to the right piriformis muscle. It is smaller than before. The differential diagnosis would include fibrotic scar tissue related to the previous surgery or a tiny mass which is responding to therapy."

Tragically, Meg was not able or was subconsciously not willing to maintain this response. For a variety of reasons, not the least of which was her reluctance to continue with healing imagery, Meg died as the result of her cancer some eighteen months later. I believe she died with peacefulness in her heart of hearts.

This chapter is dedicated to her memory and is a tribute to her courage and willingness to share her experiences with others, so that perhaps they will benefit to a greater degree.

CHAPTER TWENTY-ONE

A Review ... and the Future

People do not like to think.
If one thinks, one must reach conclusions.
Conclusions are not always pleasant.

Helen Keller

We must respect our mortality, yet be unafraid of our immortality.

In this book I have presented a wide diversity of conditions which were treated with medical hypnoanalysis. Important conclusions can be drawn, not the least of which is that the fetus is a sentient being. Another is that the severity of psychopathology and many medical disorders appears to be inversely proportional to the degree of unconditional love available to the patient in the earliest years. That is to say, the less love there is, the more likely it is that a problem may arise. Similarly, it appears that the severity of problems is directly proportional to the exposure to survival threats, be they physical, emotional or spiritual.

A few of the patients described were not outright 'cures' yet they have improved beyond what medicine and psychology appear to have achieved for those individual patients. This is not to say that medical hypnoanalysis is a better treatment but rather that it can very powerfully add to the effectiveness of medicine and psychology. All had received traditional orthodox treatment before they came to see me - as a sort of 'last resort'. I believe those who did not find total relief will, given further subconscious motivation, achieve their conscious goals. My experience has convinced me that all patients with an auto-immune disorder have an underlying subconscious reason for the disease.

A great many other problems have not been discussed such as, for example, sexual dysfunction - everything from impotence to anorgasmia and pain with intercourse; and a host of gynaecological problems - premenstrual tension syndrome, recurrent ovarian cysts, period pain ... the list is not quite endless. Many problems have their basis in an emotion/thought and are eminently treatable, many curable. This is fact.

There is the management of victims of sexual abuse and rape - the reader will appreciate that these terrible events have as their basis the unholy trinity of anxiety, fear and guilt with a large dose of toxic shame and often anger. After fifty years of medical practice, discussion and reading, I have found medical hypnoanalysis to be an extremely effective and rapid form of therapy for these patients.

There are the problems athletes present with, both in terms of injury and performance. Very often, sports people of all kinds have problems associated with an Initial Sensitising Event, a Symptom Producing Event and a Symptom Intensifying Event. If one examines the recent histories of certain professional golfers, one does not have to be a genius to see that the downturns in their careers coincided with domestic and emotional problems or a load of responsibilities imposed by sponsors. I was able to assist one golfer in bringing his handicap down from eighteen to six in just eight weeks! He was exceptional, but nevertheless he demonstrates the potential each individual has to change, or improve. Of course, he never told his friends how he did this - competitive sportsmen and women tend to keep their secrets! Yet a tragedy of South African sport is that even direct suggestion hypnosis is underutilised - we are probably sixty years behind the former Eastern Bloc countries.

The management of pain is another example. Pain always serves a purpose and the purpose is survival. In the normal course of events the body-mind alerts us to the fact that there is something wrong in our bodies which is potentially threatening to life. Such pain is usually attended to fairly promptly - the tooth abscess, the greenstick fracture of a forearm bone. When the cause is treated, the pain subsides.

Pain may be considered useful in this context and short-term severe pain is eminently treatable with traditional hypnosis in many patients.

However, the real advances are in the treatment of chronic pain, so often classified as "useless" pain by the healing professions. Many have pain as a proof of life, very often with guilt and it is **not** useless, not to the subconscious mind. The organic source of the pain may be a signal for a psychic or spiritual hurt. If not attended to, the pain will persist as the subconscious continues to remorselessly draw attention to it. There may not be any organic cause at all - hence the dismissive term "it's all in your mind", or "it's phantom pain". "It" should not be ignored. These patients can be and have been cured of their symptoms with medical hypnoanalysis.

All these and still other conditions have the same predictable ISE, a SPE and one or more SIEs. Each symptom represents a proof of life as the subconscious attempts to maintain life according to its own priorities in the order of importance: that is to say it appears that many if not most of them, have explanations in terms of learned subconscious survival responses.

There is a trend towards violent crime world-wide and remorse is infrequent. To contain this society passes laws to 'solve the problem' – history confirms this strategy is doomed to failure since no government can afford prosecute and incarcerate millions of perpetrators. Also, laws are directed at the results not the cause. As pointed out religion uses fear and guilt to change moral values - wholly ineffective because the perps subconsciously delete the guilt and it's facile to appeal to them. Remorse in these behaviours is in conflict with their proof of life! These behaviours result from a train of thought established when these people were very young indeed: the Initial Sensitising Event! It's this subconscious reaction that needs recognition and management because the subconscious cannot of its own change the train of thought.

The individuals who commit these crimes are finding a proof of life at physical, socio-economic and sexual levels because they've subconsciously accepted death at the levels of self-worth and spirit. Anger is often the energy which drives the proof of life. One could even say these acts are a function of their survival yet must be considered to be outside the law and treated accordingly. The commonest cause is the perceived absence of Love which leads to a sliding down of self-worth.

Considering the Order of Importance, it is consistently predictable that being 'dead' at level 1 and 2 – probably 3 as well – that the remorseless negative vector of violence will direct towards anti-social physical, financial and sexual behaviours. If not stalled somehow there will be a decline in society's collective conscience. How to change this direction? Awaiting a messiah is in itself a statement of our own helplessness. Perhaps a pestilence, a nuclear winter, global warming, famine, seismic disaster or an asteroid strike might induce the population to focus on a sense of humanity. An unpalatable thought is that Nature is taking its course to reduce this vastly over-populated world to manageable numbers of survival. Every organism has a growth curve which corrects itself – humanity is no different: we are at the peak right now.

Paraphrasing Prof Viktor Frankl "decent people will remain a minority; since Auschwitz we know what man is capable of and since Hiroshima we know what is at stake". Re-establishing Love at a fundamental, personal level in the nuclear family is the essential foundation. It is in this direction society and we individually should direct our best efforts.

It is also evident in the described cases that the behaviouristic psychology theories of symptoms are indeed valid - yet some comment is in order.

Firstly, behaviourism is not necessarily the whole story. It is patently absurd to assume so. Many diseases - psychological or purely medical - may have genetic predisposing factors which are crucial. Now, when there are two opposing opinions of any matter, the truth is usually to be found somewhere between … and this is true of the human condition as well. Yes, there are some purely behaviouristic problems and there are some purely genetic and physiological problems - the approach of Reductionist Theory. The majority fall between the two, with features of both to varying degrees.

It is time that both sides review their ultimate purpose and set aside more personal defence mechanisms, if indeed these play any part in the passionate battle. One has to wonder how much influence the respective fears of each group has in maintaining their own survival … research grants and the like are survival issues. I have presented a few patients' personal survival struggles which have something to say. Ultimately the opposing factions of academia come down to their respective individual personality traits. There are healers who will function far better in their calling with a scientific approach and others who will do so in a more spiritual sense. Lucky are the ones who can combine the two – even more fortunate for their patients or clients. The ultimate purpose is the concern for humanity in all its forms, in health and pain.

The behaviourists need to extend their field of vision to well before the birth of a child, for there can be little doubt that many problems revolve around the central issues of self-value and self-love, which begin in the prenatal period in the womb. That is where the personality of each individual has its foundation. This fact must now be recognised - it simply cannot be ignored. In their research, behaviourists have until now studied and documented what we know to be Symptom Producing and Symptom Intensifying Events - unaware of, or ignoring, the basic issues of the Initial Sensitising Event and the spiritual self. If one is to follow the touted "holistic approach to treatment" it is absurd to exclude the PreNatal Event. I believe that this is why the behaviourist psychotherapies have had limited success and have not achieved the results one would expect - that symptoms are modified but not eradicated. In fact, with the removal of one symptom, another is likely to emerge because of the subconscious mind's relentless compulsion to survive.

This raises an ethical issue - do we treat one symptom in isolation? The signals I receive from my own instincts are: no. My observations and instincts tell me that an alternative symptom produced by the subconscious is often worse. We need to look at the whole human being and address the **real** issues, something the behaviourists have simply been unable to effectively deal with outside of hypnosis, and the reductionists, not at all.

All health care professionals act in the best interest of their patient or client - there is certainly no intention to be the catalyst of new symptomatology. Yet this is exactly what may occur. Denial of this truth may be a dangerous path to tread ... dangerous to the patient, particularly where the JDP of guilt has played a major role in the development of the original symptom but is ignored. The subsequent symptom may well be worse.

Smoking provides the easiest example of the change of symptom. Obesity or significant weight gain is often a sequel to cessation of smoking. Some studies in the USA indicate that in the first two years after stopping smoking, the incidence of suicide rises. Aggression and impatience are another two alternative symptoms. We require some post-graduate student to do a thesis on a morbidity study of ex-smokers over a ten or twenty year period, to include **all** subsequent problems. I have a suspicion we will not like what he or she finds!

The reductionists certainly need to accept that mind and body are inseparable and that one cannot ignore the spiritual self if one is looking to achieve optimal results. Irving Gottesman of the University of Virginia, a psychologist and a leading behaviour geneticist has got it right: with regard to schizophrenia, he maintains that there is a system of predisposing genes and that the more one has of these the greater the risk of schizophrenia, given an environmental insult as the trigger.

Reductionist science seeks concrete answers one can measure. They have undertaken studies of various disorders, examining the incidence of these problems in families - utilising twins, both identical and non-identical and following them up, especially those who were adopted. They believe that if one can demonstrate similar disorders or characteristics in twins adopted to different families, this is evidence of genetic determinants.

This is of course nonsense because they exclude the fact that these separated twins shared the **same** intrauterine environment and were exposed to the **same** or similar stimuli therein but may have reacted very differently with their perceptions. In fact, many false claims on the basis of genetics have been withdrawn after initial fanfare. Examples are the 'Y' chromosome in criminal behaviour, manic depressive disorders, schizophrenia and alcoholism. The future of behaviour studies lies both in genetic determinants **and** the prenatal and early environment. Previously, the prenatal experience was dismissed out of hand or excluded, yet it is clearly a most important, critical period - this is where the seeds are sown into virgin soil.

I am particularly disappointed with many of my medical colleagues who, despite having seen their patients whom I have treated resolve their diseases, continue to ridicule and reject the evidence right in front of them. Come on people, open your minds. Your self-preservation is not helping your patients, is not providing them with options.

When an individual has experienced a loss of love in the prenatal period, that person may develop a particular emotional and behavioural response. When this person, as an adult becomes pregnant, the new baby may be exposed to similar anxieties, fears and guilt and respond in its own turn. This pattern of responses may then conceivably be perpetuated through generations ... not as a genetic phenomenon, but as a learned survival technique. Dr Michael Meaney's work and many others in the field of epigenetics indicate that as a result of these stressors, the genetic expression itself may be altered. It is possible that over several generations a physical genetic adaptation may occur.

It therefore may become very difficult to distinguish between the two schools of thought.

While the researchers continue the good work in their respective laboratories, those involved at the coal face - actually treating patients or clients - need to be aware of the positive aspects of both schools. Hand-in-glove co-operation is required, because such complementary management of a patient can only be to the patient's advantage. That is of course why we are here.

There are a few peripheral issues we can address, applying the information in this book. The first may not seem a critical issue, yet we should be aware of the possibility of harm.

The issue of anti-smoking advertising is an area that may need review. Yes, the goals are obviously noble, but the methods used closely follow those of a dictatorial parent or rigid, didactic religious instruction: **fear** and **guilt** are the emotions utilised. These methods make smokers feel guilty about injuring their children and their unborn babies, and strike with fear with the suggestion of cancer and heart disease. Smokers are compared with narcotic addicts. One should be aware that the comments on each pack of cigarettes constitute **suggestions**, which are duly noted by the subconscious of each buyer. Such open and subliminal suggestions may ultimately result in a response which I submit is often the opposite of the advertising's intention! The anxiety, fear or guilt reproduces the emotions of the original threat in many smokers - their subconscious minds are still compelled to respond in some way. There can hardly be a smoker who is not aware of the health risks. Very few people will consciously and deliberately spend a lot of money to cause him- or her-self injury. Clearly, this behaviour is not under their conscious control ... it is subconscious, otherwise they would not do it. To achieve a healthy transition we should be addressing the real issues, not acting after the horse has bolted.

The strategic approach to drug addiction must recognise the emotional and spiritual issues described in this book. The late Dr Sylvain de Miranda argued for lifestyle education for twenty years in this country and it is gratifying to see that this is now being slowly introduced. It is a start, but we need a far greater effort to manage the problem at its source: *ab initio* unconditional love and effective management of the crises in life. The latter are not even recognised by most people - the circumcision at eight days of age; the tonsillectomy at four. These are just two major events which to the child may be life-threatening issues, which we have not recognised and have therefore ignored.

Obviously the issue of abortion is quite horrifying to me. I am not claiming to be a saint - quite the opposite. I was a member of one hospital's termination of pregnancy committee and I was sympathetic to the problems of many women. However, I resigned my position after the first prenatal regression I did. There was no possible way I could reconcile the two, no way could I continue to condone or advocate termination. I could no longer play God.

This may or may not be the only country in the world which sanctions the murder of the insularly helpless yet cognizant foetus, while safeguarding the human rights of a convicted murderer. This profound paradox is one of the great ironies of the new South Africa. I have seen one advertisement for "safe abortion". The obvious question that needs asking is: "Safe for whom?" Certainly not the baby. There is now a move in the United Kingdom to recognise abortion as a birth control method …

The United Nations announced the principle that "The life of an individual human being begins with conception and ends with death. The right to life is the most basic of all rights, and belongs also to the foetus in the mother's womb." The Declaration of the Rights of the Child in 1959 continues: "the child by reason of its physical and mental immaturity needs special safeguards and care, including appropriate legal protection before as well as after birth."

One of the arguments for termination of pregnancy is that legalised abortion will save many lives at risk from back street abortions. Yet, the latter still happens. The cold hard truth is that we **collude** with this behaviour. Legalised abortion also negates the development of self-discipline, and allows people to maintain immature thought, emotion and behaviour. It perpetuates the Ponce de Leon Syndrome. It is a known fact that some of these patients do **not** learn from the experience. Some reappear for second and third abortions, and the problem is such that sterilisation of these women is considered. I believe that simple statistics will reveal that we kill far more babies by legal abortion than the number of women who lose their lives to back street abortionists.

The reader of this book, understanding the reality of the foetus' environment and its reactions to it, will have to agree that abortion cannot be condoned at any level, morally or spiritually. It is a barbaric practice in my opinion. It is an example of the power of lobbyists and government and the use of the Law of Man which contradicts the life principle itself in favour of short-term goals, be they socio-economic or political. If this was the result of ignorance in the past, such justification can no longer apply.

I do not for one moment believe that women who have had an abortion escape without negative emotional and spiritual effects. I have treated the effects of guilt in enough of these patients, which always resulted in a serious psychological or medical disorder, some of them catastrophic. Even the Dis-social Personality Disorder patients, who have suppressed guilt very deeply, are significantly affected.

I have demonstrated that many of the symptoms and symptom complexes we have involve just one subconscious imperative: survival and that the highest priority is Love.

Without love, there is no reason to live and one dies in a spiritual sense, entering an existential void. Further, at a subconscious level, one may believe that one has died at a physical level. Preceding this acceptance of death is the phenomenon of fear - the attempt by the subconscious to avoid that death. Should there be no finalisation of this threat because of immature logic or unconsciousness, that fear is translated into a chronic low-grade fear which we call anxiety: the fight or flight response when there is no actual threat present. The real source of this later anxiety is the original powerfully perceived survival threat. This fear can be released once the realisation of survival has taken place in the subconscious.

Guilt brings with it the fear of spiritual death - the fear of rejection by mother or father or the potential loss of God's love. As this love of God is the energy of one's spirit, the result of loss is a seemingly bottomless pit of darkness - a contributor to the major depressive disorders, psychosis and often life-threatening physical disease.

The patient may sink so deep into this darkness that he or she may develop the conviction that he or she is no longer a worthy human being and may thereafter consistently create unhappiness in life. He or she may simply dissociate from life, entering his or her own world, safe from threat but no longer capable of taking an active productive and fulfilling part in life. Some become self-destructive and leave this world physically - by disease or suicide - conforming their body image to that already established in the subconscious mind.

The tragedy is that each of the above is based on a faulty belief system directly attributable to the Initial Sensitising Event. It is this belief which must be sought, confronted and altered with the careful guidance of the therapist.

The absence of this love - real or perceived - is the major contributing factor to strife on this planet, individually and globally. On the grand scale there are political groups, socio-economic groups, religions and cultures acting out the result of their component members' individual

Initial Sensitising Events and their struggle to survive. Striking parallels exist in the history of some individuals and world history —this is logical because the history of mankind is dependent on its individual members' responses.

I can imagine the best of worlds in which each pregnant mother has as her basis of living a firm and immovable self-love, supported by a husband who can similarly stand up and react to the world in a calm and confident manner ... parents with faith in love. Their children will surely have the best of opportunities in life, with the unconditional acceptance of their being. Events such as birth and death would be managed far more easily with such a sound foundation. Their potential would more easily be realised.

It would be wonderful if every child somewhere in the teenage years had the benefit of medical hypnoanalysis so that they can achieve the internal peace required for the foundation of their own children's personality.

Given all the other healthy aspects of civilisation - a positive religious belief, education and primary health care, I wonder ... I wonder what the world would look like four or five generations down the line? Or ten?

That may be an unrealistic vision. OK, humour me. And remember, "what can be imagined, can be achieved."

Ask the Wright brothers.

Ask James Joyce.

SOURCES, REFERENCES AND GLOSSARY

Ader R, Cohen N. Behaviourally Conditioned Immunosuppression & Systemic Lupus Erythematosus. *Science. March 19; 215: 1534-1536.*

Anderson MC; Green C. Supressing unwanted memories by excutive control. *Nature* 2001; 41: 131-134.

Begley S. Faster than What? *Newsweek June 19, 1995; 44-45.*

A report on Raymond Chiao and his colleagues' work at UCLA, Berkley.

Begley S. Holes in those Genes. *Newsweek January 15, 1996 ; 41.*

A report on Michael Meaney's work at McGill University.

Berg PS. Miracles, Mysteries and Prayer. *New York : Kabbalah Centre Books, 1993.*

Blozik E; Rapold R; Eichler K; Reich O. Epidemiology and costs of multiple sclerosis in Switzerland. Dove Press. Nov 2017; Vol 2017:13; 2737-2745. https://www.dovepress.com/article 35402.t76921097

Boslough J. Stephen Hawking's Universe. *Glasgow : Fontana Collins, 1989.*

Bryan WJ Jnr. The Walking Zombie Syndrome. *Journal of the American Institute of Hypnosis. 1961; 2 (1): 38-50.*

Capra F. The Tao of Physics. *London: Flamingo, 1992.*

Coville WJ, Costello TW, Rouke FL. Abnormal Psychology. *New York : Barnes & Noble Inc; 1968.*

Croswell K. To Kill a Galaxy. *Astronomy Dec. 1996; 36-41.*

Flamsteed S. Crisis in the Cosmos. *Discover March 1995; Vol 16 No 1: 66-77.*

Flanagan LF. Beginning Life. *London: Dorling Kindersley 1996.*

Frankl VE. The Doctor and the Soul. *New York: Vintage Books 1986.*

Frankl VE. Man's Search for Meaning. *London: Hodder and Stoughton 1987.*

de Girolama G, Reich JH. Personality Disorders. *Geneva: World Health Organisation 1993.*

Grof S. The Holotropic Mind. *San Francisco: Harper Collins 1992.*

Hawking S. A Brief History of Time. *London: Bantam Books 1994.*

Horgan J. Eugenics Revisited. *Scientific American June 1993; 93 - 100.*

Janov A. The Primal Scream. *London: Abacus 1973.*

Kaku M. Hyperspace. *Oxford: Oxford University Press. 1995.*

Klein DF. False Suffocation Alarms. *Paper: 9th SA National Psychiatry Congress 1996.*

Laing RD. Knots. *Harmondsworth, Middelsex: Penguin 1970.*

Leckman J; Mayes IC; Cohen DJ. Primary maternal preoccupation revisited: circuits, genes and the critical role of early life experiences. *South African Psychiatry review,* 2002; 5: 4-12.

Lesney MV. Gene Farming and the Biopharmaceutical Revolution. *Analog 1993; CXIII(10):60-75.*

Lindberg NE, Lindberg E, Theorell T, Larsson G. Psychotherapy in Rheumatoid Arthritis - a parallel-process study of Psychic State and Course of Rheumatic Disease. *Z Rheumatol 1996 - i:28-39.*

Lu, S. Erasing bad memories. American Psychological Association; *February 2015, Vol 46, No 2:42.*

Lueck R. Psychoneuroimmunology and Hypnoanalysis. A summary of the AAMH Fall Conference. *Medical Hypnoanalysis Journal 1992; Vol VII(4).*

Marais E. The Soul of the Ape. *Johannesburg: Jonathan Ball 1990.*

Modlin CT. Medicine and the Spiritual Self: Reflections. *SA Family Practice Vol 14, No 11; 483-490.*

Modlin CT. The Cause and Treatment of Conduct and Antisocial Personality Disorder. *Medical Hypnoanalysis Journal June 1991; Vol VI (2): 69-76.*

Modlin CT. Clinical hypnosis and psychoneuroimmunology. *Continuing Medical Education Journal. Jan 2008; Vol 26, No. 1; 8-11.*

Modlin CT. "I don't remember dying": a case study of the resolution of chronic pain utilising Medical Hypnoanalysis. (2012). *South African Journal of Psychology, 42, (2), 182-190.*

Motz L. The Universe - Its Beginning and End. *London: Abacus 1977;241-2: 305-7.*

Murray L, Cooper PJ, Stein A. Editorial. *BMJ SA Edition 1993; 1(5).*

Obsessive Compulsive Disorders. *In Psychiatry in Practice 1995;*

Vol 2, No 1: 40-44.

Ornish D. Can Lifestyle Changes Reverse Coronary Artery Disease? *Lancet July 21 1990.*

Plotsky PM; Meaney M. Early post-natal experience alters hypothalamic corticotrophin-releasing factor mRNA, median eminence CRF content and stress induced release in adults. *Molecular Brain Research 1993; 18:195-200.*

Pepper, Frank S. 20th Century Quotations. *Sphere Books: London; 1987.*

Ritzman TA. The Cause and Treatment of Anxiety. *Medical Hypnoanalysis Journal 1988; Vol III (3): 95-115.*

Ritzman TA. Guilt. *Medical Hypnoanalysis Journal 1993; Vol VIII(1): 10-18.*

Ritzman TA. Depression and the Nature of God. *Medical Hypnoanalysis Journal Nov 1982; 129-139.*

Scott JA Snr. The Handbook of Brief Psychotherapy by Hypnoanalysis. *Winfield : Relaxed Books; 1996.*

Siegel B. Love, Medicines and Miracles. *Arrow Books: London; 1988.*

Siegel B. Living, Loving & Healing. *The Aquarian Press: London; 1993.*

Sharpe M, Hawton K et al. Cognitive Behaviour Therapy for Chronic Fatigue Syndrome. *BMJ 1996; No 5 Vol 4: 608-12.*

Simonton OC, Henson R. The Healing Journey. *Bantam Books: New York; 1992.*

Spiegel D, Kraemer HC, Bloom JR, Gottheil E. The effect of Psychosocial Treatment on Survival of Patients with Metastatic Breast Carcinoma. *Lancet October 14 1989; Vol II (8668): 888-891.*

Steiner R. Reincarnation and Karma. *Vancouver: Steiner Book Centre, 1977.*

Sternberg EM, Gold PW. The Mind-Body Interaction in Disease. *Scientific American. Mysteries of the Mind: Special Issue Vol. 7 No1 1997; 8-15.*

Strean HS, Freeman L. The Severed Soul. *St Martin's Press 1990.*

Thomas PK. Editorial - The Chronic Fatigue Syndrome: What do we Know? *BMJ. Sept 1993; Vol 2: 4-5.*

Wong J, Holdaway I. Galactorrhoea. Causes, Diagnosis and Management. *Therapeutics Feb 1997; Vol I No. 8: 37-40.*

Zeilik, Gaustad. The History of the Universe. *In Astronomy: The Cosmic Perspective; 2nd Ed New York; Wiley 1990.*

Zelling DA. Multiple Sclerosis. *Medical Hypnoanalysis Journal Sept 1994; Vol IX No 3: 98-109.*

Zelling DA. Spiritual Being. *Editorial Medical Hypnoanalysis Journal 1990; Vol V (2): 44.*

I would like to thank the Editor of the SA Family Practice Journal for permission to reprint two diagrams from an article I wrote which the Journal published.

GLOSSARY

ISE   Initial Sensitizing Event
SPE   Symptom Producing Event
SIE   Symptom Intensifying Event

The subconscious diagnoses:

PNE   Pre-Natal Experience: perceptions of the fetus and its reactions to the environment during the intra-uterine life

IDP   Identity Problem: A loss of the sense of Meaning, purpose and belonging as the result of a perceived or actual absence of Love.

DES   Death Expectancy Syndrome: the expectation of death – the fundamental emotion of Fear. This is commonly generated during birth, known as the Birth Anoxia Syndrome or with the separation from maternal love at birth known as the Separation Anxiety Syndrome. May also occur *in utero*.

WZS   Walking Zombie Syndrome: the subconscious acceptance of death either physically and/or with the idea that life is no longer worth living.

PDL   Ponce de Leon Syndrome: An emotional immaturity in which an individual becomes stuck in childhood and locking in an immature response to life events in adulthood.

JDP   Jurisdictional Problem of Guilt: A self-imposed judgement and self-punishment resulting from an actual or perceived wrong-doing in an attempt to avoid divine punishment after death; as if suffering in this life will prevent divine rejection.

The Order of Importance of subconscious survival

The subconscious priorities of Survival, from least to most significant:

7. Sex	.....	Species survival
6. Territory	.....	Socio-economic survival
5. Food }		
4. Water }	.....	Physical survival
3. Oxygen }		
2. Self-esteem	.....	Ego or Mind survival
1. Self/**Love**/Soul/God	.....	Spiritual survival

www.ingramcontent.com/pod-product-compliance
Lightning Source LLC
Chambersburg PA
CBHW021351210526
45463CB00001B/63